PRAISE FOR
Natural Beauty Reset

"This book is essential reading for any woman trying to navigate the choppy waters of healthy living. Hormonal health is the key to a happy and healthy life and this book helps make sense of how to bring things into harmony."

—Pedram Shojai, OMD, *New York Times* bestselling author of *The Urban Monk*

"If you want to feel better inside and out, start with this book! Dr. Cates is an empathetic, expert guide through the delicate complexities of women's hormones and beliefs around beauty—you *will* learn something new."

—JJ Virgin, *New York Times* bestselling author of *The Virgin Diet*

"Want to look and feel youthful, radiant, and gorgeous? With Dr. Cates as your guide, you can discover how to transform yourself from the inside out. In this book, she'll guide you to becoming the beautiful, confident, happy woman you want to be."

—Dr. Kellyann Petrucci *New York Times* bestselling author, *Dr. Kellyann's Bone Broth Diet*

"Dr. Cates has been my trusted source for skincare for many years. Her new book will help people reclaim their beauty and get healthy along the way!"

—Alan Christianson, NMD, *New York Times* bestselling author of the *Thyroid Reset Diet*

"Health and beauty are deeply connected, and *Natural Beauty Reset* encourages beauty by prioritizing physical, mental, and emotional health. At a time when there are so many conflicting messages around women's health, hormones, and happiness, Dr. Cates's knowledgeable guide is a truly refreshing read!"

—Izabella Wentz, pharmacist and *New York Times* bestselling author of *Hashimoto's Thyroiditis*

"If you care about your health, your beauty, and your overall quality of life, you must read my favorite book of 2022, *Natural Beauty Reset*. As an integrative physician and women's hormone expert, I know what it takes for women to optimize their health, so I enthusiastically recommend this book, as it addresses the major topics related to hormonal balance, blending science with great practical advice, both holistic and delicious!"

—Dr. Felice Gersh, MD, board certified in OB/GYN and Integrative Medicine

Natural
BEAUTY
RESET

Natural BEAUTY RESET

The 7-Day Program to
Harmonize Hormones and
Restore Radiance

Dr. Trevor Cates

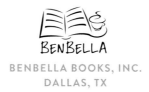

BENBELLA BOOKS, INC.
DALLAS, TX

BenBella Books, Inc.
10440 N. Central Expressway
Suite 800
Dallas, TX 75231
benbellabooks.com
Send feedback to feedback@benbellabooks.com

BenBella is a federally registered trademark.

Printed in the United States of America
10 9 8 7 6 5 4 3 2 1

Library of Congress Control Number: 2022935023
ISBN 9781637741269 (print)
ISBN 9781637741276 (ebook)

Copyediting by Ruth Strother
Proofreading by Amy Zarkos and Michael Fedison
Indexing by WordCo Indexing Services
Text design and composition by Faceout Studio, Paul Nielsen
Cover design by Oceana Garceau
Cover and interior photography by Adam Finkle/ajfphoto.com
Printed by Versa Press

Special discounts for bulk sales are available. Please contact bulkorders@benbellabooks.com.

I dedicate this book to the sisters in my life. This includes those who are biological as well as the sisters who are part of my community, and that includes **you**. Remember, you'll **always** be beautiful!

CONTENTS

Foreword xi

Introduction 1

PART I.   The Root Causes 6

CHAPTER 1.   Hormones, Cycles, and Rhythms 9

CHAPTER 2.   Gut, Bugs, and Your Radiance 19

CHAPTER 3.   Mood and Memory 25

CHAPTER 4.   Time to Restore 31

CHAPTER 5.   Food, Habits, and Seasonal Changes 37

CHAPTER 6.   Too Toxic 43

PART II.   The 7-Day Natural Beauty Reset Program 51

CHAPTER 7.   Food, Movement, Mindset, and
              Skincare for the Seasons 52

CHAPTER 8.   Fall Reset (September, October, and November) 60

CHAPTER 9.   Winter Reset (December, January, and February) 79

CHAPTER 10.   Spring Reset (March, April, and May) 99

CHAPTER 11.   Summer Reset (June, July, and August) 116

CHAPTER 12.   Personalizing the 7-Day Natural Beauty Reset 134

CHAPTER 13.   Natural Beauty Reset Recipes 150

Resources 234

Acknowledgments 235

Notes 236

Index 244

FOREWORD

Being healthy, beautiful, and radiant is as much an inside-out process as it is an outside-in one. It is a balance between what you put inside your body, what touches your body on the outside, and your overall quality of life—achieving optimal health is a holistic process. Among many other things, your health will determine how you age and how you look as you age, which is why I love the inherent and learned wisdom of Dr. Trevor Cates in the pages that follow. Her approach goes far beyond how to get glowing skin; it helps the reader understand how this glow comes from an overall sense of balance, and provides them with the tools and knowledge to achieve this. It helps them understand their own bodies, enabling them to look and feel their best.

An incredible piece of the puzzle is certainly our nutrition plan. As a physician for over twenty-five years, I have found that women of all ages, and especially around menopause, do better when we change up our eating habits throughout the year. We do have seasons for a reason. In *Natural Beauty Reset*, Dr. Cates includes nutrition plans for fall, winter, spring, and summer. I appreciate this strategy. It reminds us, every season, to adjust to our environment, and incorporate seasonal healing foods and recipes to support our immune system, hormonal balance, mood, memory,

and skin. Tuning our bodies to the shifting seasons in this way helps us reconnect not only with our environment, but with our own bodies. It gives us a sense of well-being and natural radiance that you just can't achieve with skincare alone.

I love the line from the Broadway musical *Annie*: *You're never fully dressed without a smile.* When we think about beauty, isn't it true that a smile makes a face more beautiful? Joy and happiness bring a genuine smile. In *Natural Beauty Reset*, with its comprehensive deep dive into the root causes of our physical struggles—from external stress to internal hormonal imbalances—Dr. Cates acknowledges that we cannot just look beautiful and radiant; we need to *feel* it.

In my professional experience, I know this to be true: while interventional therapies like stem cells, peptides, and laser treatments have helped make progress in patients feeling more beautiful and healthy, these external solutions account for less than 10% of what it means to actually *be* healthy. True vitality comes from multiple sources: nourishing our body with the right foods at the right times and the correct proportions, incorporating regular physical activity into our lives, maintaining good relationships, and a careful consideration of what we are putting on our body are all crucial components of our health.

What we apply on our skin is absorbed into our skin and gets into our system; it is all connected. By the time a woman leaves the house in the morning, it's estimated she has put over 180 chemicals on her body. Many of these chemicals are hormone disrupting. In fact, we are exposed to a multitude of toxic chemicals before we are even born. A study performed in 2004 looked at toxic chemicals found in newborn babies' umbilical cord blood. Two hundred eighty-seven external chemicals were identified in the blood, 208 of which were known to cause birth defects and abnormal development in animal studies, 217 of which were found to be toxic to the brain and nervous system, and 180 of which were known to cause cancer in humans and animals. Pesticides, herbicides, toxic compounds, waste from burning garbage and gasoline, and so many other toxins that we inhale or seep into our skin daily affect our health and can be at the core of many of the hormone imbalances we struggle with. Toxic exposures and hormone disruptors are a significant and underappreciated cause of health problems, especially considering the hundreds of thousands of chemicals in circulation.

In the European Union, they've banned over 1,350 chemicals; however, in the US that number is less than 100. In my work as a gynecologist and hormone expert, I recognize that to heal, revitalize, and reenergize our bodies, we must get to the root cause of our issues. And that is a key component of aging gracefully and radiating beauty. It is essential we take a pause, and really take a good look at everything we are exposed to daily and how it all impacts our health. Choosing organic, safe, nourishing products and essential oils will alleviate our system from a tremendous toxic burden. This book will empower you to identify the potentially harmful substances you're exposed to every day and make informed choices about finding safe alternatives.

As we age, we begin to truly value the importance of our health, and begin to understand how the quality of our lives, our moods, our mental state, our immune strength, our energy, and our relationships impacts that health. An old Arabian proverb says, *When you have your health, you have a thousand wishes; when you don't have your health, you have but one.*

Dr. Trevor Cates's new book, *Natural Beauty Reset*, guides you through this process of achieving balance, radiance, and overall health with clarity and practical, easy-to-incorporate tools to completely support you on your journey. This resource, along with a healthy diet and lifestyle, is truly the magic recipe to healthy aging and radiant beauty.

—ANNA M. CABECA, DO, FACOG, triple-board-certified OB/GYN, and bestselling author of *The Hormone Fix*, *Keto-Green 16*, and *MenuPause*

INTRODUCTION

When I was eleven years old, I used to spend hours on end staring at myself in a multifaceted mirror in the bathroom of my grandparents' house. I wasn't dwelling on every angle of my appearance out of vanity. Instead, I was lonely and wanted company. As odd as it may sound, the reflections looking back at me became friends whom I could talk to and share the secrets I often kept bottled up inside.

Despite feeling isolated, I had what many people would consider an idyllic childhood. My parents, sisters, and I lived on an organic farm with plenty of nourishing food and love to go around. But neither of those advantages changed the fact that I felt I didn't belong.

You see, my family was—and is—full of what society considers beautiful people. My eldest sister was a model in New York City. My other sister was on the homecoming court and the one that every girl at school, including me, wanted to be. My mother also was stunning and dabbled in modeling, and my father captured women's eyes and hearts with his smile and charm. In my eyes, they were perfect—and I was the ugly duckling of the family.

When I looked in the mirror at myself, I thought I was an impostor. So I tried my best to disappear, tending to spend my time quietly while self-quarantining in my room or getting lost in nature. I watched my family excel in life and was truly proud of them all. I didn't get praise for my looks the way my sisters did, but one day when I came home with a report card showing all A's at school, to my surprise, I got extra attention. So, that's when I decided I wasn't "beautiful," but I was smart. So, I focused my efforts on my studies.

What I didn't realize then but now know is that I, too, was (and am) beautiful. We *all* are. And we will *always* be beautiful. We just are looking in the wrong place for confirmation: mirrors. But mirrors show what we alone are perceiving of ourselves on the outside and don't reflect our true beauty inside.

As I approach my fiftieth birthday, I see myself clearly. This realization wasn't instant. Pain and heartache encouraged me to change my perspective gradually. As the poet Rumi so eloquently put it, "The wound is the place the light enters you." And when I learned to heal my internal wounds on my healing journey, the light flooded in.

Being beautiful is not about being perfect, but it does involve restoring balance. It starts with harmonizing our health, including our hormones, and adjusting our mindset. This was the answer to the secret I had been searching for all of those years while studying my face in the mirror.

I know that I'm not alone in my history of insecurity and self-doubt—and I hope other women who relate can muster the courage to follow suit and find harmony and balance in their lives. When we address our vulnerability with kindness and honesty, we can quiet our inner monsters and overcome society's warped messages around beauty.

Over the years, I've heard from thousands of women in my clinics and programs, as well as hundreds of women experts I have interviewed for my podcast and docuseries. The personal stories these women relayed have revealed that regardless of age, income, physical characteristics, or talent, every woman questions her lovability and beauty at some point. We are not alone in our struggles! But what we also share is that when balance has been restored in our bodies—including harmonious levels of hormones and neurotransmitters—our perceptions of ourselves shift, and ultimately our true beauty shines.

Through these conversations, I've also learned that women face challenges unique from men, and that these challenges have the potential to affect our self-worth and self-perception. For instance, many women tend to work around the clock—at work and at home—often caring for our loved ones. We get up early and stay up late, and, sadly, we give ourselves little time to rest. We try to squeeze in time to eat and work out but are frustrated when we gain rather than lose weight. We often feel isolated, though we're rarely really alone.

We're trying to do everything but still feel like we're failing because we stretch ourselves thin and put everyone else first. We often feel that we are not smart enough, not pretty enough, not thin enough, not [fill in your word here] enough. And with all of the chronic stress that results from these habits, we feel burned out and overwhelmed. Many of us also develop physical issues that impact the way we look and feel—from acne breakouts, period problems, and unhealthy weight gain to exhaustion, fogginess, and pain.

To find the answers to our struggles, we often turn to male-centered research (because that's the majority of what's being funded) and media that uses filters and airbrushes to enhance the appearance of already beautiful models and make us feel even more ashamed and misunderstood. But the answers are actually within us and closely connected to our body's innate wisdom. We must first stop living out of sync with our rhythms because it weakens our hormonal function, immunity, digestion, and detoxification capabilities. When we pay attention to our female biochemistry, address the root causes of whatever is ailing us, and tailor our self- and healthcare to our feminine needs, we can tap into our bodies' full potential. Then we realize how truly powerful we are.

According to Merriam-Webster, beauty is "the quality or aggregate of qualities in a person or thing that gives pleasure to the senses or pleasurably exalts the mind or spirit."[1] Put differently, beauty, by definition, is all about an individual's external attributes from someone else's perspective. Over time, factors like magazines and social media, plus the beauty industry, have led us to form attitudes around what that perspective should be.

It's no wonder many women use makeup to cover "flaws" or fork over hundreds or thousands of dollars to a plastic surgeon to alter our appearances. Nor is it a surprise that we are compelled to slap on a skin-perfecting filter on social media photos. And neither is it a wonder that many of us buy the same old "superfoods" year-round, thinking they're a silver bullet for glowing skin. (Hint: looking and feeling great is more complex than that!)

You might be thinking: *But I* want *to be the woman who turns heads when I set foot into a room!* For this book, I ask that you first look within because seeking external validation is not where you'll find solace and success. Embracing *natural* beauty takes a 360-degree approach—one that starts from within.

But before we go any further, let's get one thing straight: this is *not* an anti-beauty book! As a woman, I realize the notion of giving up beauty routines altogether is unrealistic. Not only are self-care and pampering considered routine in so many of our daily lives, but at their core, these rituals are integral to our well-being.

With my Natural Beauty Reset, you don't have to give up your beauty routine—I'm simply encouraging you to rethink it.

In this book, you will learn how hormonal imbalances and common self-care practices are a barrier to achieving physical and emotional beauty and how to restore your health and harmony naturally. This solution includes food but goes further. We are hungry for something that can't simply be found in kale or mac and cheese. It also goes beyond simply believing we are beautiful. Mindset is key, but without internal balance, it is hard to realize our full potential. Ultimately, after reading this book you will have the inspiration and tools necessary to rekindle your innate beauty now and for years to come.

My clients and I are living proof that this approach works. Today, I feel more vibrant and confident than ever, knowing that restoring balance in a new way helps me see and feel what my eleven-year-old self did not. I want that harmony and confidence for you, too.

Although I've been practicing holistic medicine for over twenty years, the light bulb moment that inspired this program happened after I published my last book, *Clean Skin from Within*, a *USA Today* and Amazon bestselling book. The book focuses on taking a natural inside-out approach to treating skin conditions such as acne, rosacea, and eczema with personalized skincare and dietary advice. After the book was published, I heard from women who still had questions about the connection among their hormones, skin, health, and aging. I've always known beauty is beyond skin deep, but I realized then that many women weren't attaining their goal of clean, glowing skin because they hadn't set the proper foundation first. That is, they weren't looking inward, nor were they cognizant of the natural rhythms and cycles around them that beg for connection.

(Side Note: She/Her—While I use the words woman, women, she, her throughout *Natural Beauty Reset*, this book is really about empowering you to make healthier choices and can be enjoyed by everyone regardless of gender and sexual identity. When I discuss female sex hormones, those sections will be most relevant to anyone who has a uterus and ovaries. However, if you do not have your uterus and

ovaries or are no longer cycling, it is still important to understand the hormones discussed within this section because they do impact your health. Some people who identify as women may not have the biophysical makeup being explored in this book. If you identify as trans or nonbinary, or are taking estrogen or testosterone as you undergo gender transition, you may have unique health and well-being needs. However you identify yourself, or wherever you are in your gender journey, understand that much of this book will apply to you. If you are undergoing gender transition, follow the recommendations of your healthcare provider about your individualized hormonal needs.)

Making Adjustments with the Seasons

Tried and true healthy habits are important for our general health. However, living a healthy life from a holistic perspective must involve more than simply grabbing to-go meals from the health food aisle at the grocery store, attending a quick yoga class at the gym, and using skincare with the word *natural* on the label. We want to be more discerning and avoid the marketing traps that can trick us with false promises of being healthy, natural, or stress-free. It's time to dive deeper and understand how and why we need to make these health choices so we can set more meaningful intentions.

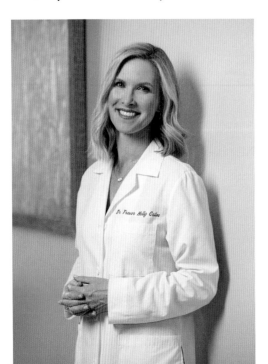

Our skin, stress levels, nutritional needs, and hormones cycle through significant changes throughout the year, so why are we following the same diet, skincare routine, and exercises every day? Our needs change each season and so should our approach. That's why in the 7-Day Natural Beauty Reset program, you'll find a set of distinct changes with each season that support optimal nutrition and gut health. This approach allows our bodies to reconnect with the way we were designed, with the dynamic shifts of nature. The result? Authentic beauty with optimized health and radiance.

You will receive year-round foundational guidelines and learn how to effectively adjust them with each season. You'll learn my seven-day plan for fall, winter, spring, and summer, with seasonal modifications for:

❀ **Food**
❀ **Movement**
❀ **Mindset**
❀ **Skincare**

All four aspects are crucial for lasting beauty that glows from the inside out.

The discussion of natural rhythms has been explored since the dawn of womankind, but it's time to marry traditional wisdom from credible scientific research with a truly holistic and restorative program for the modern woman.

We still want our self-care practices and pampering, so I will share how you can maintain your routine while also restoring internal balance and hormonal harmony.

This book is designed to help you regain your power mentally, emotionally, and physically. Ultimately, your body is your home—you are the one in charge. My goal is to help you restore your body to the happiest and healthiest haven, so you'll have the ability to radiate natural beauty. Your glow has always been there. I'm simply guiding you toward a fresh reveal.

PART I

The Root Causes

"When did you realize you are beautiful?" I asked her.

At the question, Amy's eyes widened with her mouth agape. Then she smiled, her gaze gleaming with certainty. She wasn't used to being called beautiful, but when she heard those words, something deep within her stirred, and she knew the statement was true.

The aforementioned anecdote comes from a ten-part docuseries in which I interviewed over fifty experts of various ages on women's health and hormones. When I witnessed this particular interviewee's reaction, my gut wrenched in empathy. So often, as women, we doubt our beauty. But when we dig deep, we can surface our truth. Specifically, I have learned that when we are attuned to natural rhythms and our hormones become balanced, our beauty is unveiled, sparkling bright for the world to see.

Attaining a healthy mindset is an important step in this mission. After all, how we perceive ourselves tends to reflect what may be happening inside. But we can't simply force our minds to embrace the notion that we're beautiful. Sometimes, the root cause is physiological. Put

differently, we can't simply change our mindset when our bodies are out of sync.

Also instrumental is how we choose to nourish our bodies, whether and how we move, what we're applying to our skin, whether we're in touch with our breathing, and taking time to unwind. These are the tenets that provide a foundation so many women are lacking in order to look—and feel—beautiful.

Modern-day beauty tools, technology, and even takeout can be convenient and easy, but they tend to distract us from the keys to feeling and appearing truly beautiful. In particular, these habits have caused us to lose connection with the innate wisdom found in seasons, cycles, and rhythms. As a result, issues with mental health, digestion, and nutrition can result. These afflictions tend to show up on our skin and impede the ability for us to see our true beauty.

Modern technology also affects hormonal balance. The smartphone, for instance, has a glowing blue light that interferes with production of melatonin, a hormone that is critical for quality sleep. Hormones rule our skin, mood, and health more than most women realize. We need

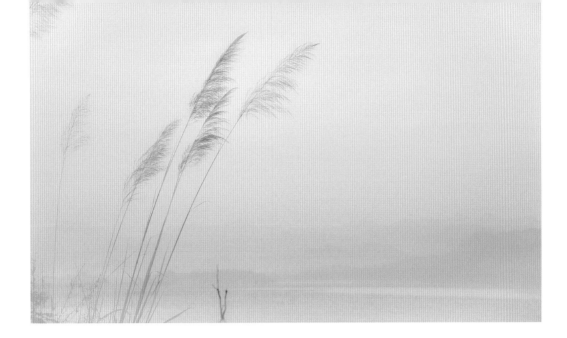

our hormones working well to truly feel uncaged and beautiful.

I do not know a woman in the Western world over the age of thirty who has not faced skin issues, hormonal imbalances, and emotional ups and downs during her lifetime. The connection between these goes deep, and yet most doctors treat them separately.

Rates of depression and anxiety were higher during the pandemic,[2] and depression is more common in women than men.[3] Yet doctors typically prescribe antidepressants without addressing the hormonal root causes that contribute to so many women feeling emotional and out of sync.

For acne and other skin issues, doctors often treat these superficially with topical steroids. Women commonly receive prescription birth control pills for acne and other hormonal issues, like irregular menstrual cycles, even when they're not sexually active, but these conventional treatments come with side effects and do not address the true underlying cause.

These are the women who have come to me: women who are confused, emotional, and out of sync. While their symptoms may have improved temporarily with conventional interventions, their symptoms return and sometimes worsen. And many develop side effects such as gut issues, nutritional deficiencies, and hormonal and neurochemical imbalances.

The solution to realizing our authentic beauty is right in front of us—found in the rhythms, wisdom, and healing of nature. I will share my Natural Beauty Reset solution, including meal plans, recipes, and other lifestyle advice in part II. But first, it's important to understand how root causes may prevent us from seeing and feeling our innate beauty.

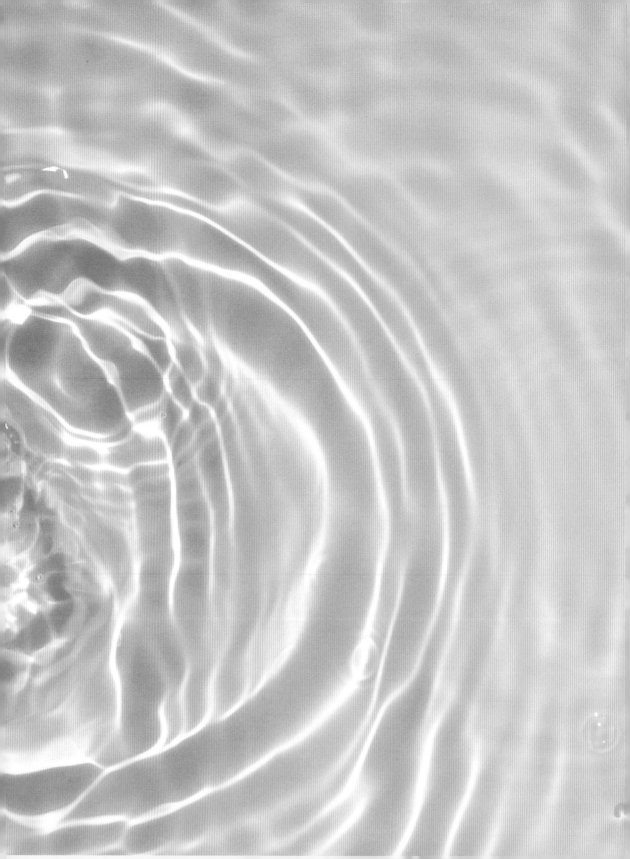

CHAPTER 1

HORMONES, CYCLES, AND RHYTHMS

Think of hormones as musical instruments and your body as a symphony. Each instrument must play its part perfectly—including being at the right volume, rhythm, pitch, melody, and tone—to create a balanced and beautiful-sounding song. If even one instrument is playing too loudly or too softly or is out of key, for example, your body's hormonal system will be thrown off-balance. And that imbalance will show up in and on your body. Put simply, hormones, skin, mood, and health are intertwined.

Externally, possible signs of hormonal imbalance include dryness, acne, rosacea, and premature fine lines and wrinkles. Internally, they include impaired

metabolism, mental focus, memory, cognition, mood, sleep, energy, fertility, and sex drive. Hormones also play a role in cardiovascular health, bone growth, and blood sugar regulation. Overall, hormones help us be more resilient, both mentally and physically, and have more time and energy to do epic things.

One challenge is that our hormones change as we age. The delicate balance that our bodies are so adept at also starts to evolve. There are a variety of hormones at play here, and some may surprise you.

If you've seen symptoms of hormonal imbalance in yourself, don't worry—I'm here to help you learn how to address these issues naturally. I will cover how to restore balance in part II, but first I will explain the problem so that the solution will be crystal clear.

Things We Do That Disrupt Hormones

Believe it or not, many of your everyday habits—including those related to eating, sleep, stress management, and exercise—can disrupt hormones. Certain medications such as birth control pills can throw hormones for a spin, too, and lead to nutritional deficiencies and gut issues that further worsen the problem. Chronic stress, such as from a draining job or relationship troubles, has the potential to disturb hormones, decrease quality of life, and may eventually contribute to mood disorders.

Another major factor in hormone disruption can be found in the ingredient list of some personal-care products. Many of these items contain endocrine-disrupting chemicals (EDCs), which are absorbed through the skin into the bloodstream and can potentially wreak havoc on our endocrine system. According to the Endocrine Society,[4] EDCs are associated with fertility issues, early breast development, breast cancer, prostate cancer, thyroid disease,[5] neuroendocrine problems, obesity, and cardiovascular disease.

A critical step in reducing exposure to EDCs is to be picky about what we put on our skin. For example, avoid using oxybenzone (found in popular chemical sunscreens), parabens, and synthetic fragrances because they have been linked to hormone-disrupting effects. I will share a full list of ingredients to avoid in chapter 6, but for now, know that you're better off avoiding EDCs.

Key Hormones and How They Impact Our Health

Hormones impact us much more than most people realize, affecting mood, sleep, sex drive, energy, weight, metabolism, skin, bones, cardiovascular system, joints, and digestion. As a doctor who helps people understand their hormones' behavior—and then helps people get back on track—it's hard for me not to geek out here! I invite you to do the same. It's fascinating stuff!

Before we get into Hormones 101, grab a notebook. The following information will be more helpful when you start observing your own hormonal shifts and patterns. As you read through this chapter, you may be able to pinpoint the specific hormones influencing your health (details that will come in handy in part II). Also, notice which hormones tend to change on a daily, monthly, and seasonal basis, as these will be important at that point, too.

Here are some of the main hormones that impact the way we look and feel:

- Estrogen
- Progesterone
- Testosterone
- Thyroid hormones thyroxine (T4) and triiodothyronine (T3)

- Dehydroepiandrosterone (DHEA)
- Cortisol
- Insulin
- Melatonin
- Leptin and ghrelin
- Oxytocin

ESTROGEN

Estrogen is the hormone that gives us curves and fertility, but it also plays a role in protecting the brain, bones, skin, and heart. We make estrogen in our ovaries, adrenals, fat cells, and other tissues.

Estrogen levels decline as we age, especially after forty and as we approach menopause. There are other times in a woman's life, such as before puberty and just after pregnancy, when estrogen levels decline. Also, women who have had their ovaries removed go through what's called surgical menopause. Even throughout a cycling woman's month, estrogen levels dip at certain times, which can impact mood. Women's estrogen levels may also be higher in summer months compared to winter.[6]

Low estrogen makes the skin drier, less elastic, and more fragile. It can also cause bone loss, hot flashes, insomnia, mood changes, night sweats, infertility, and vaginal dryness. On the other hand, high estrogen comes with its own set of problems. Women who are pregnant or on birth control pills generally have higher estrogen levels and are more prone to melasma (hyperpigmentation). There are also many women who experience what is often called estrogen dominance, where estrogen is not metabolized properly or when progesterone starts to decline starting around age thirty-five, or both, leading to excess estrogen compared to progesterone.

The key with estrogen, as with all hormones, is balance, which changes at different times of a woman's life and monthly cycle. But keep in mind that while symptoms of estrogen imbalance are common, they're not optimal. And there are ways we can restore balance naturally. When we are free of symptoms like hot flashes, irregular cycles, and vaginal dryness, as well as signs on our skin of melasma to premature aging, we can feel more beautiful inside and out. Beauty is our natural state—and we deserve to feel vibrant and healthy at every stage of our lives.

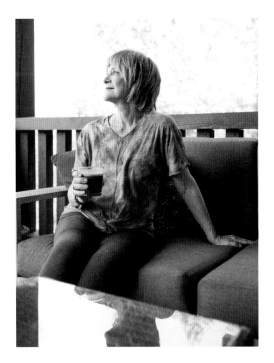

PROGESTERONE

Progesterone is mostly produced in the ovaries and plays an important role in an array of bodily functions, including fertility, appetite, fat storage, and mood. Not to mention, it provides protective effects for our skin, bones, breasts, and uterus. When balanced, progesterone helps us feel calm, but when it's low, we can feel irritable and experience sleep trouble.

Progesterone helps counterbalance estrogen, aiding a healthy menstrual cycle. So when our progesterone levels are low, unpleasant period symptoms such as irregular and/or heavy bleeding, hot flashes, and night sweats can also happen.

TESTOSTERONE

Testosterone is not only a hormone for men. Women make and need it, too, just in a different way. In women, testosterone is made in our ovaries and adrenal glands. This hormone helps keep our bones strong, protects our brain, aids energy maintenance, and regulates mood. When testosterone is low, we may lack drive and confidence.

Skin-wise, testosterone stimulates the sebum-producing glands, which are important for protecting skin with natural oils, but overproduction can lead to acne. Age-related hormonal changes, such as those experienced during puberty and menopause, may affect testosterone and metabolism, leading to oily or breakout-prone skin.

Unfortunately, even adults without a history of teenage acne may develop blemishes as a result.

The active metabolite dihydrotestosterone (DHT) is the main culprit for androgenic side effects in women such as unwanted facial hair growth, hair loss on the scalp, and acne. These are some of the potential symptoms of polycystic ovary syndrome (PCOS), an underdiagnosed endocrine disorder in women. PCOS is characterized by higher than normal levels of androgens, including testosterone.

Yet too little testosterone isn't ideal. Symptoms of low testosterone may include reduced sex drive, brain fog, mood changes, fatigue, thinning and dry skin, muscle loss, and a reduction in bone mineral density, which can increase the risk for fractures.[7] Groups of women at risk for insufficient testosterone include those who are on the pill and those approaching or experiencing menopause. To support healthy testosterone levels, exercise and eat a healthy diet with plenty of protein. Find more ways to support testosterone levels in chapter 12.

THYROID HORMONES
THYROXINE (T4) AND
TRIIODOTHYRONINE (T3)

Thyroxine (T4) and triiodothyronine (T3) are the two main thyroid hormones released from the thyroid gland. T3 is the active form, which comes from T4. Our thyroid hormones support metabolism, energy, and mood.

With low levels (clinically diagnosed as hypothyroidism), you may have fatigue, constipation, hair loss, and weight gain. Low thyroid in women is also associated with irregular menses, infertility, and miscarriage. An underactive thyroid can lead to a dry, coarse complexion and a reduced ability to perspire.

On the other side of thyroid imbalance, an overactive thyroid, or hyperthyroidism, can cause symptoms such as weight loss, rapid heartbeat, increased appetite, and irritability, as well as warm, sweaty, and flushed skin.

If you're having symptoms or think your thyroid hormones are out of whack, talk with your doctor about thyroid testing. The tests to ask for are thyroid stimulating hormone (TSH), Free T3, Free T4, reverse T3, and thyroid antibodies. Testing can also reveal if you have thyroid antibodies, which indicates an autoimmune thyroid condition such as Hashimoto's thyroiditis.

In the wintertime, levels of active thyroid hormone T3 tend to be higher than in the summer, suggesting a seasonal difference.[8] This makes sense because thyroid hormones help with thermoregulation, keeping us warm during the winter. Keep this in mind if you have a thyroid condition.

DEHYDROEPIANDROSTERONE (DHEA)

Produced in the adrenal glands, DHEA plays a role in energy, memory, body fat, skin aging, and sex drive, and levels decline with age. DHEA converts to estrogen and testosterone, which means it's our primary source of these hormones when our ovaries stop producing them after menopause. Keep this in mind around perimenopause because if your adrenal glands are taxed by producing too much cortisol, they will have a harder time making adequate levels of DHEA.

CORTISOL

When you're stressed, your adrenal glands release the hormone cortisol. Too much cortisol can lead to symptoms such as sleeplessness and excess belly fat. But too little cortisol is not good, either, as it helps support our immune system, regulate inflammation, and balance blood sugar and blood pressure. Cortisol also helps us wake up in the morning!

Surges of this hormone due to a highly stressful situation may cause increased sebum production, triggering acne and amping up inflammation, thereby making almost any skin condition worse. Chronically high cortisol levels can worsen skin conditions, including acne, eczema, rosacea, and vitiligo. A high level can also lead to sugar cravings—and eating excess sugar increases inflammatory skin issues.[9] So you may get caught in a vicious cycle.

Experiencing chronically imbalanced cortisol levels can leave you feeling "tired but wired." If you've noticed weight gain around your middle section or you're experiencing fatigue, insomnia, or sugar cravings, you may need extra support to balance your cortisol levels.

Even when balanced, cortisol levels tend to change throughout the day, which is important to remember because your energy and mood will fluctuate accordingly. Some simple adjustments can help you feel your best, such as breaking a sweat in the morning (when cortisol levels are supposed to be at their highest) and going for a short walk, taking a power nap, journaling, or meditating at around 4 PM, when cortisol rises again.

Cortisol levels can change seasonally, as well, with studies showing higher concentrations in winter and early spring, and lower levels in summer.[10] The great news is there are many practical and straightforward steps you can take to ease the effects of stress on your body all throughout the year on your journey to natural beauty.

INSULIN

Insulin is released from the pancreas and helps the body regulate blood sugar, which is crucial for our metabolism as well as our overall health. It allows glucose (sugar) in our bloodstream (from the foods we eat) to be taken up and used as fuel. If we have too much sugar and our blood sugar is high, insulin signals the body to store the excess in the liver. Insulin levels appear to change with seasons, with lower levels in the winter and higher levels in the summer.[11]

When blood sugar swings after we eat excess sugar, such as candy and pastries, and refined carbohydrates, such as potato chips and white bread, the risk for insulin resistance (where cells cannot sense insulin, and blood sugar stays elevated) increases.

Diabetes is one disease that occurs when the body doesn't make enough insulin or doesn't use insulin properly. It's been estimated that over 470 million people will have prediabetes (where blood sugar levels are elevated but not high enough to be considered diabetes) by the year 2030.[12] The American Diabetes Association states that up to 70 percent of people with insulin resistance will develop type 2 diabetes. Yet many of these cases can be prevented by making lifestyle changes.

Improper insulin function in the body can get in the way of your natural beauty. When sugar stays in the bloodstream, rather than being ferried to cells the way it's supposed to for energy, glucose (blood sugar) binds to proteins, which is called glycation, in the body. Two of those proteins are essential for healthy, naturally youthful skin: collagen and elastin. Glycation can accelerate the formation of wrinkles and sagging skin.

When insulin isn't working properly, your energy levels and weight may also fluctuate. And if you develop type 2 diabetes, you may face increased thirst and appetite, tingling sensations in your hands and feet, fatigue, irritability, headaches, frequent urination, and increased infections.

Getting your insulin, fasting glucose, and hemoglobin A1c tests can help determine if you have insulin resistance. I recommend aiming for your fasting blood sugar to be in the 85 to 90 mg/dL range. Even though the normal range is below 100 mg/dL, it's better to be proactive and start making changes in your lifestyle before your levels creep up above 100 mg/dL. You also don't want your blood sugar to be too low, so if your blood work shows fasting blood glucose below 70 mg/dL, talk with your healthcare provider about whether you need to be monitored for hypoglycemia, or low blood sugar, because that may cause dips in your energy level and other health concerns.

MELATONIN

When was the last time you got a good night's sleep and woke up to a glowing, refreshed face? Send your thanks in part to melatonin, the so-called sleep hormone.

When it's dark, the pineal gland in the brain releases melatonin. On the other hand, when it's light (whether artificial or natural), the pineal gland inhibits melatonin. It stands to reason that this hormone is designed to help us feel sleepy when the sun sets, and it peaks around 2 AM to 4 AM to help us stay asleep. Melatonin gradually decreases after 4 AM, and when the sun rises, our levels drop and the sleepiness wears off, triggering wakefulness.

Seasonal changes in light—such as longer summer days and shorter winter days—affect melatonin production. Mammals, including humans, have higher melatonin levels in winter compared to summer. In addition to light, exposure to cold temperatures appears to increase our production of melatonin.[13]

Besides sleep, melatonin[14] provides other benefits, including protection against neurodegenerative diseases such as Alzheimer's and Parkinson's, certain types of cancer, mood disorders, and PCOS.[15] Interestingly, melatonin potentially has the ability to reach every cell in the body, creating a wide array of protective benefits and relaying communication about the circadian rhythm throughout the body.

There are even melatonin receptors found in the uterus, and some scientists believe the hormone may help with the management of labor.[16] There is also evidence that melatonin changes with our cycles.[17] Melatonin appears to be at its highest level right before menstruation, and levels decline as we age and get closer to menopause.

LEPTIN AND GHRELIN

If you've ever struggled to control your eating habits or modify your weight, leptin and ghrelin were involved.

Fat cells make leptin, which helps curb appetite—that is, it increases a feeling of fullness after eating. Some people have leptin resistance, which can make weight maintenance challenging. Ghrelin is a hormone primarily released in the stomach and increases appetite. Simply put, ghrelin helps encourage eating to avoid starvation, and leptin tells us to stop when our bodies are satisfied. But this harmonious relationship between these hunger and satiety hormones isn't easy for some people, such as those with obesity, genetic predispositions for food cravings,[18] poor lifestyle choices, and mood and metabolic issues.

Interestingly, research has shown higher sensitivity to leptin in the winter compared to the summer, when ghrelin levels tend to dip, which may explain why our hunger changes seasonally.[19] Specifically, the data suggests that we may have less of an appetite in the winter than the summer. Knowing about leptin and ghrelin helps us be more mindful of our hunger and modify our eating habits with the seasons.

OXYTOCIN

There's even a hormone associated with cuddling.

Oxytocin is sometimes called the love or cuddle hormone because of the sense of bond we feel after its release. Childbirth, breastfeeding, and sex trigger oxytocin production, but so does simple, everyday touch such as with hugging. Women typically have higher levels than men, and it has both physical and emotional effects, impacting our social behavior, connection with others, and feelings of trust.

Even with technology at our fingertips, it's important to connect with others for hugs, hand-holding, massages, and other forms of touch to help keep cortisol in check and stave off stress.[20] This balance is key to looking and feeling your best.

These are just a sample of the numerous hormones that impact our health as women, and are important to understand in order to achieve natural beauty. Too often, women are given antidepressants and sleep aids instead of addressing hormonal

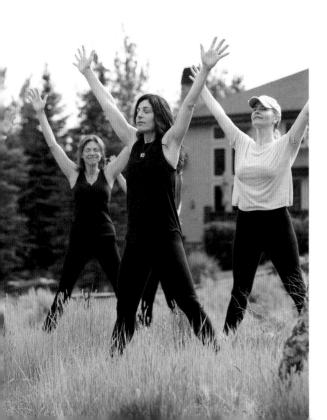

imbalances. Or they're put on birth control pills for acne. Hormonal imbalances are often overlooked at a typical doctor's appointment for women.

Ideally, when our hormones are balanced, we wake up feeling rested before our alarm goes off (thanks to a healthy elevation in cortisol). We don't need coffee or naps because we have energy throughout the day (hello, balanced blood sugar, and thank you, insulin). We don't need acne treatments or concealers (because our androgen levels are balanced). At the end of the day, we start to feel sleepy (drop in cortisol), and when the lights go out (melatonin rises), we fall asleep without night sweats or hot flashes (thank you, progesterone and estrogen).

We are free of migraines and moodiness before our periods (as estrogen and progesterone are balanced), and our periods are Goldilocks just right (not too heavy, and not spotty or absent). When we snuggle up with our partner and feel connected (boost in oxytocin), we have a great sex drive and ability to orgasm without being obsessed about it (due to balanced testosterone) and plenty of vaginal lubrication (thanks to adequate estrogen).

All of the above happens in a perfectly balanced hormonal state. But most of us do not have this every day, and some women have never experienced this balance. But that's okay. Our hormone levels evolve, which is 100 percent normal. The key is to become balanced and resilient so on the days we are not feeling harmonious,

our bodies are able to bounce back. In part II, you'll learn about the Natural Beauty Reset that will help you achieve both balance and resilience.

For now, I want you to know how these hormones play a role in your health and mood so you don't think it's all in your head, that you should suppress symptoms, or that there's no hope. There are solutions, which you'll find in part II in the seasonal plans. And you will know how to specifically hone in on any remaining hormonal imbalances by answering the questions in chapter 12.

Start thinking about which of your hormones may be out of balance and how that might be impacting your health. Just because a woman has insomnia, for example, doesn't just mean she needs melatonin.

Case Studies

To provide an example of how a single symptom can be caused by a variety of hormonal imbalances and the importance in finding the specific hormone out of balance, here are three patients who came to see me with insomnia. I will explain more about treatment options in chapter 12.

JULIE AND THYROID

Julie was a thirty-two-year-old woman who was experiencing fatigue, weight gain, and dry skin. With insomnia being her primary symptom, it would be easy to assume her melatonin levels were off and that fatigue and weight gain were natural consequences of sleep deprivation. And we could have credited her dry skin to living in the dry climate of Park City, Utah. Testing revealed the truth. In fact, melatonin hadn't been the problem at all. Rather, feeling too cold at night (a result of underactive thyroid) had been keeping her awake. After I gave her thyroid support, balancing her thyroid hormones, and prescribed lifestyle and dietary changes, her temperature normalized, and she began to snooze soundly. Problem solved!

SARA AND PROGESTERONE

Sara was a forty-six-year-old woman who mentioned she was feeling sad and anxious before her periods and had occasional night sweats. When I ran a hormone panel, it revealed her progesterone levels were low. With a treatment plan that included progesterone support with diet changes, herbal supplements, and bioidentical hormones, her insomnia and night sweats disappeared, and her mood was much more even throughout the month.

TERESA AND CORTISOL

Teresa was a fifty-three-year-old woman who struggled to wake in the morning and began noticing weight gain around her midsection despite being athletic. At night, she struggled to unwind and fall asleep. With testing, we discovered her evening cortisol levels were high. With supportive care to manage her stress and balance her cortisol, her insomnia disappeared.

ONE RESULT, MULTIPLE CAUSES

As you can see from these examples, one symptom such as insomnia can have a variety of hormonal causes. All of these women reported that their doctors prescribed sleep medication. However, if they had resorted to taking a sleep aid, they would have missed out on addressing the root causes of their sleep trouble, and their other symptoms would have continued. Down the road, these hormonal balances could have created additional health challenges. That's why identifying the problem hormone through testing is so critical.

While correcting hormonal imbalances can feel overwhelming, rest assured that the adjustments and reset program in part II will put your body's hormones in sync and your mind at ease.

CHAPTER 2

GUT, BUGS, AND YOUR RADIANCE

Getting back in touch with nature also means getting a bit dirty. You may be thinking: *but I* like *my hand sanitizer, bleach, and scented antibacterial body wash.* I hear you! Improvements in hygiene and sanitization have been positive in many ways, not least of which is that they have helped prevent infections. And anyway, who doesn't want to feel clean and live in a hygienic environment? The problem is we've gone too far, and the potential consequence of living in the highly sanitized society of today—one that has, frankly, become germophobic—is an imbalanced microbiome.

Microbiome refers to the balance of microorganisms such as bacteria, protozoa, viruses, and fungi of various areas of the body. That includes the gut, the mouth, the respiratory and urinary tracts, the vagina, and the skin. Scientists began researching the microbiome in the 1990s, with the gut being the biggest area of interest, but other microbiotas of the body have been gaining more attention in recent years. If you want the CliffsNotes, know this: a healthy gut microbiome has a direct effect on health overall, and your hygiene habits may very well be disrupting the delicate balance of bacteria in yours.

Perhaps your response is: but I don't have bloating, constipation, diarrhea, gas, or stomach pain; my gut is perfectly healthy! Unfortunately, that's a myth. An imbalanced gut microbiome can show up without these pesky digestive issues.

The good news is that the awareness of the microbiome and the possible harms of living in a too-clean world is shifting. That's all thanks to research and people like you who are asking questions.

What Is the Gut Microbiome?

Your gut microbiome in particular affects several parts of your health, including the harmony of your hormones, your mental health, your biological age, and your skin.

Your gut microbiota started developing when you were in your mother's womb, and then it continued to evolve with every point of contact you've had with microorganisms. Birth method, nursing approach, medications, diet, pet exposure, and hygiene practices are all examples of factors that can affect the gut microbiome early on. These exposures have laid an important foundation for your health.

Here are just a few of the things our gut microbes (bugs) do for us:

- Keep harmful bacteria and other germs in check
- Produce vitamins such as vitamin B_{12}, thiamine, riboflavin, and vitamin K
- Minimize inflammation in our bodies
- Support a healthy immune system
- Help regulate our hormones
- Aid in digestion of food
- Support our ability to metabolize drugs
- Impact our brain health

- Play a role in maintaining a healthy weight
- Improve insulin sensitivity (helping with blood sugar balance)
- Help protect against certain chronic diseases, including diabetes, fibromyalgia, irritable bowel disease, inflammatory bowel disease, cardiovascular disease, and obesity
- Influence the health and appearance of the skin

Here are some of the major factors that disrupt our gut microbiota:

- Antibiotic therapy, birth control pills, and proton pump inhibitors
- Overzealous hygiene practices
- Food intake with little diversity of produce and low fiber
- Cigarette smoking
- Altered intestinal mobility (constipation or diarrhea)
- Artificial sweetener consumption
- Altered pH (too high)
- Excess protein and sugar intake

When it comes to maintaining good health, a healthy gut microbiome is one that is balanced. We don't want too many of certain microbes, and some microbes we simply don't want. But the right balance can help support our bodies' digestive, immune, cardiovascular, metabolic, mental, hormonal, nutritional, and inflammatory status. The end result is greater homeostasis and less disease.

We need a healthy gut microbiome for optimal digestion and absorption of nutrients from our food, but if our digestive tract lining is damaged, we also need to address it.

While you've likely already heard the term *leaky gut*, *leaky skin* is a more novel concept, yet it is one worthy of your attention, especially during these times of heightened hygiene practices. Leaky skin (the external epithelium) is connected to leaky gut (the internal epithelium).

Our bodies are beautifully designed to send nutrients from the food we eat out to every cell in the body to provide nourishment, which is why our bloodstream is connected to our intestinal cells. The tiny cells in our small and large intestines let through very small molecules, like vitamins and minerals, into the bloodstream, while keeping out harmful microorganisms and substances that don't belong in our bloodstream. To assist with this, our intestinal cells have junctions that bind the intestinal cells tightly to each other. When we eat, these tight junctions get a signal to open up and let nutrients through, but then they close so nothing else can permeate the barrier. Leaky gut happens when these tight junctions are compromised, and instead of being able to close back up, the channels are always open, allowing undigested food particles or harmful microorganisms to get through into the bloodstream. The body naturally triggers inflammatory pathways to fight invaders in the bloodstream. Once

our tight junctions are compromised and we have leaky gut, chronic inflammation will follow—harming our gut and overall health.

I'm going to explain how to address this issue in part II, but for now, let's turn our attention to the skin microbiome.

What Is the Skin Microbiome?

The skin microbiome promotes the natural lipid barrier and skin immune system, which helps restore and promote vibrant-looking skin. The skin microbiome is the term used for the trillions of bacteria, fungi, protozoa, and viruses that live on our skin, and that includes one thousand different bacteria species and almost eighty different fungi species.[21] An estimated one million bacteria inhabit each centimeter of our skin. But the makeup of these bacteria remarkably vary by skin region and by individual person. Lifestyle, environment, hygienic practices, diet, age, and sex can impact the composition of the skin microbiome.

From the inside out, our gut microbiome impacts the skin microbiome.[22] There are short-chain fatty acids that arise from the fermentation of fiber in the gut (from the foods we eat) that influence the makeup of the bacteria on the skin.

Consuming high-fiber and prebiotic-rich foods is one way to promote the growth and activity of healthy gut microorganisms. Examples of prebiotics include garlic, leeks, onions, chicory root, dandelion greens, oats, barley, and apples. Taking probiotic supplements may also support the skin barrier function, several studies suggest.[23]

What you consume is not the only factor that can affect the skin microbiome—what you apply topically matters, too. Antibacterial agents, for example, can kill off not only harmful bacteria but also beneficial microorganisms that live on and protect the skin from breakouts, eruptions, and premature aging.

Now, let's take it back to high school chemistry. Remember pH? It's a measure of how concentrated hydrogen ions are and can tell us how acidic or alkaline a solution

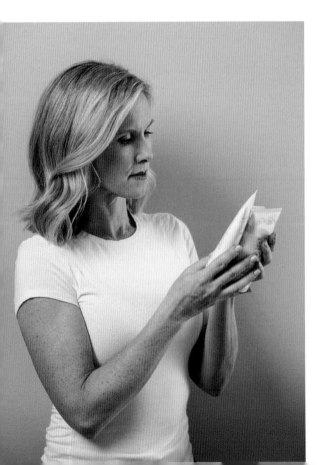

or surface is. The surface of human skin has a natural pH level of about 4.0 to 4.5, making it mildly acidic.[24] This value helps keep the skin's microbiota in balance; a more alkaline pH (anything over 7.0) kills or disrupts that balance. Even water's pH of 7.0 is too high for skin. After rinsing with water, rebalancing the pH to a mildly acidic level is important. Many common skincare products, including cleansers, serums, moisturizers, and OTC topical medications, have a pH of 5.5 and higher, which can dry out skin and make it more prone to infections and premature aging.[25]

Ideally, our skin would always maintain the target pH. But certain beauty rituals, hygiene practices, and environmental factors can disrupt the skin barrier. Because it would be unrealistic to live in a protective bubble and totally eliminate exposure to environmental factors, the best we can do to help the skin return to and maintain a healthy pH is to carefully select our skincare products. I learned about this when I dug into the research to create The Spa Dr. skincare line.

The ideal pH of a skincare product is between 4.6 and 5.4, and the ingredients that go into the product determine this value. Various natural ingredients, such as citric acid, may reduce a formula's pH to that mildly acidic range. Not all skincare products are made with mild acidity in mind. You also don't want the skincare products to be too acidic, which is below 4.5. In addition, certain oils, such as argan kernel oil, can help restore resilience to the acid mantle while at the same time imparting luminosity and preventing dryness.

Cleansing is one of the biggest mistakes people make in their skincare routine. Most cleansers have a pH that is too high (over 5.5) and contain ingredients that strip the skin of its beneficial oils. Start with a mildly acidic plant-oil-based cleanser, such as The Spa Dr.'s Step 1 Gentle Cleanser, even if you have skin prone to oiliness. Then you can follow with an antioxidant-rich serum, such as The Spa Dr.'s Step 2 Antioxidant Serum, that nourishes your skin, and a moisturizer and face oil, such as The Spa Dr.'s Step 3 Enriched Moisturizer and Step 4 Glow Boost, respectively, that hydrate and protect your skin.

In addition to promoting an ideal skin pH, it's imperative to support the skin's microbiome by using natural actives that help restore balance. Topically used probiotics appear to adhere to human keratin and prevent biofilm formation, indicating they may help maintain a healthy skin microbiome.[26]

Research shows that topical products containing prebiotics or probiotics, or both, may help the skin by modulating the immune system.[27] They also appear to improve skin rejuvenation.[28] More research is unfolding on the use of probiotics in skincare, but this is particularly important for those of us with dermatologic conditions such as acne and eczema, as well as individuals with dry, sensitive, and reactive skin.

My fifty-one-year-old patient Rebecca experienced imbalances in her skin when she switched her skincare products. She came to see me for perimenopausal symptoms and mentioned that her skin felt dry and dull, and wrinkles were suddenly becoming more prominent. A month after changing her skincare products to The Spa Dr.'s more mildly acidic natural skincare line, she noticed an improvement in the hydration and smoothness of her skin.

The skin and gut microbiotas help provide protection from the external environment. When well balanced, both can help minimize oxidative damage and exposure to allergens, as well as repair damaged barrier functions. (Oxidative damage happens to cells and tissues when the production of free radicals exceeds the body's ability to counteract their damaging effects with antioxidants.) If we lose beneficial microbes, we lose their protection, and it can show up on our skin as blemishes and premature aging.

What Should I Know About the Vaginal Microbiome?

In addition to the skin and gut microbiotas, we have many other areas around the body where microorganisms reside and impact our bodies' functions. An important area for women is the vaginal microbiome.

Imbalances in the microbiota of the vagina, such as overgrowth of *Gardnerella vaginalis* (the dominant bacteria in bacterial vaginosis), have been linked to an increased risk of pelvic inflammatory diseases, miscarriage, poor wound healing (such as post-surgery), and increased risk for sexually transmitted infections.[29] We now know that bacteria are not all bad. In fact, having bacteria in the vagina is essential for women's health. The issues arise when there are imbalances in the vaginal flora.

DIGGING DEEPER

Did you know that in 1892, the beneficial bacteria *Lactobacillus* was originally called *Doderlein's bacillus* after the man Doderlein, who isolated this bacteria from vaginal specimens of healthy pregnant women? Thankfully, it was renamed! Isn't it interesting that a male researcher would have the nerve to name a woman's vaginal bacteria after himself? However, some things still haven't changed . . . The bacteria *Gardnerella vaginalis* was identified by Gardner and Dukes who described this organism as the primary cause of white discharge syndrome.

Various factors play a role in the vaginal microbiome, including sex hormones (such as estrogen levels), hormonal birth control methods, sexual behavior (such as new sex partners), hygiene practices, smoking, and diet.[30]

Because everything in the body is intricately connected, many of the lifestyle choices we make for supporting our gut microbiome also support the vaginal microbiome. When we restore balance to our natural state, it's amazing what our bodies can do! More on this in part II.

CHAPTER 3

MOOD AND MEMORY

"Where did I put my keys?" "What is her name again?" "Why did I walk into the kitchen? I can't remember what I came here to get!"

Sound familiar?

Throughout our lives, we have forgetful moments. And that's normal. But at times, we may notice an increase in these mental slips. Life stages that cause hormonal fluctuations, such as pregnancy and perimenopause, may also influence our cognition.

Lapses in memory can be frustrating and embarrassing, triggering stress—and that doesn't do the brain any good. Yet it can be comforting to know there are physiological reasons for forgetful and moody moments, and they're tied to our hormones and neurotransmitters. When we restore balance to these systems, we can improve both our mood and our memory.

Forgetfulness was my patient Jessica's main concern when she came to see me. A forty-seven-year-old schoolteacher, she was concerned her poor memory was negatively affecting her job. When I dug into her medical history and symptoms list, it became clear that her chemical messengers were at the root of her concerns.

As Jessica and many of my other patients have discovered, ongoing stress, lack of sleep, hormonal imbalances, poor nutrition, and certain medications can trigger or worsen neurochemical imbalances. Genetics are an underlying factor, too, but the good news is that we have more control over our genes than we used to believe. That means how we choose to live in our bodies can impact genetic expression—essentially, to turn our genes on and off, resulting in certain health outcomes. I'll share my blueprint for this in part II, which has helped Jessica and my other patients.

In the previous chapter, we explored the relationships between the various microbiotas of a woman's body. The research now connects brain health with our gut health, calling it the gut microbiota–brain axis.[31] The idea behind this is that the gut microbiota affects the development and functioning of the brain. The research has associated imbalances in the gut microbiota (gut dysbiosis) with neurological conditions such as anxiety, depression, autism spectrum disorder, and multiple sclerosis.

Certain neurotransmitters such as serotonin, gamma-aminobutyric acid (GABA), and acetylcholine have been isolated from bacteria within the human gut and appear to play a role in the gut–brain axis.[32] It appears that stress can disrupt the gut microbiome, and dysbiosis can affect behavior. Issues with the microbiota gut–brain axis negatively impact[33] the hypothalamic-pituitary-adrenal (HPA)[34] axis and vice versa. The HPA axis refers to the interaction among the hypothalamus, pituitary gland, and adrenal glands.

Genes, early life stress, and current stress levels can all affect the HPA axis. When we experience stress, neurotransmitters trigger the activation of the HPA axis in the hypothalamus. This causes the release of hormones that activate the anterior pituitary gland, which in turn stimulates the release of hormones such as cortisol from the adrenal glands. These effects are connected with the hormonal imbalances that we discussed in chapter 1.

How Hormones and Neurotransmitters Compare

Both hormones and neurotransmitters are chemical messengers that carry signals from one part of the body to another. The difference is that hormones are made by endocrine glands, whereas neurotransmitters are produced by the nervous system.

There are more than forty neurotransmitters—some prime examples include dopamine, GABA, epinephrine, norepinephrine, and serotonin. Let's explore these neurotransmitters so you can see the importance they can play in our mood and memory and how our lifestyle (including medications and supplements we take) can influence them.

* Dopamine
* GABA
* Norepinephrine and epinephrine
* Serotonin

DOPAMINE

Remember the last time you felt really good? Dopamine was probably involved. This neurotransmitter affects how we experience rewards (such as food, sex, shopping, and anything else that brings us pleasure) and how we think and plan accordingly. It's involved in our drive (both sexual and overall motivation), learning, memory, and motor control.

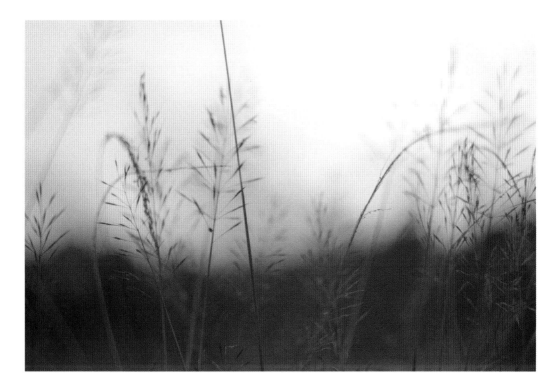

When dopamine increases, our focus sharpens and motivation and overall happiness rise, so in a balanced place, dopamine can aid productivity and boost mood. However, it also can lead to addictions and not-so-ideal lifestyle choices. Nicotine and alcohol, for example, activate the dopamine receptors causing a quick rush of dopamine, making smoking and drinking habit-forming. But over time, we need more dopamine to get the same feeling, which may increase the risk for addictions and unhealthy behavioral patterns. This feeling can also make us act more compulsively in search of that dopamine high. Dopamine-related disorders include alcoholism and other drug addictions.

When dopamine is low, we may feel less alert and motivated and have difficulty concentrating. Low levels can also cause challenges with focus, coordination, and movement. The amino acid tyrosine and its relative phenylalanine, called neurotransmitter precursors, can be used to enhance dopamine production.

GABA

Think of GABA as your internal promoter of peace. As a neurotransmitter, GABA works by blocking impulses among nerve cells in the brain, which helps have a calming and neuroprotective effect.[35] Glutamate, the precursor to GABA, has the opposite role, and instead will excite.

Low levels of GABA have been linked to anxiety, depression, insomnia, aggressive behavior, and chronic pain.

Factors that play a role in poor GABA activity include genetics, poor sleep, inadequate diet, stressors, certain medications, and gut issues. Estrogen[36] tends to suppress GABA, while progesterone[37] and its metabolites tend to facilitate its production.

GABA occurs naturally in certain foods, and studies show that GABA as a supplement may help improve mood, memory, and sleep. In addition, the amino acid L-theanine, which occurs in green and white tea, can have a similarly calming GABA-like effect.

A fermentation process with the bacterial strain *Lactobacillus hilgardii* is used to make GABA supplements. These supplements may work directly through the blood–brain barrier or via the gut.[38] Magnesium binds to GABA receptors and activates them, which may explain why magnesium also has been shown to improve quality of sleep.[39] Meditation and movement such as yoga also appear to help improve GABA activity.[40]

NOREPINEPHRINE (NORADRENALINE) AND EPINEPHRINE (ADRENALINE)

These two hormone-neurotransmitter hybrids are crucial for our survival. They act as the main neurotransmitters of our bodies' sympathetic (fight-or-flight) nervous system. They act as both hormones and neurotransmitters to help the body and brain respond to various emotional and physical stressors. Both affect our heart, blood sugar, and blood vessels in response to stressors.

Low levels have been associated with anxiety, depression, migraines, hypoglycemia, and sleep disorders. High levels can cause anxiety, high blood pressure, headaches, and heart palpitations. Chronic stress and poor nutrition are contributing factors to these imbalances.

SERATONIN

Serotonin is dopamine's sibling in that it also helps you feel happy, not to mention calm and focused. This neurotransmitter is derived from the amino acid tryptophan and is found primarily in the intestines, brain, and blood platelets.

The most commonly prescribed antidepressants are selective serotonin reuptake inhibitors (SSRIs). These medications block the reabsorption of serotonin into neurons, which increases the availability of serotonin as a neurotransmitter and subsequently boosts mood. Common side effects of SSRIs include nausea, headaches, insomnia, agitation, dizziness, blurred vision, suicidal thoughts, and problems with sexual performance. Too much serotonin activity in the brain, such as with serotonin syndrome from taking too many SSRIs, can cause symptoms such as anxiety, tremors, confusion, high fever, and rapid heart rate.

Because serotonin is also found in other areas of the body, it plays other roles there as well. For example, in the intestines, serotonin impacts appetite and digestion. It's also a precursor to melatonin, so it plays a role in sleep.

Taking serotonin supplements or eating foods like bananas that contain naturally occurring serotonin won't boost your mood because this neurotransmitter is not able to cross the blood–brain barrier. That means we have to rely upon boosting our serotonin levels in other ways.

Thankfully, there are ways to increase serotonin without simply relying upon drugs.[41] For example, meditation, light therapy, and regular exercise may help naturally increase serotonin levels in the brain. Taking tryptophan or its relative, 5-HTP, will increase serotonin levels. Both can cross the blood–brain barrier: 5-HTP more readily, while tryptophan requires a small amount of carbs to help it across.

※ ※ ※ ※ ※

Understanding the role these neurotransmitters play in our mood and memory helps us grasp the importance their balance plays in our health and well-being. Using medications to mask symptoms may provide temporary relief but can also come with side effects, and medication does not address the true root causes.

In part II, the Natural Beauty Reset program will help you restore a healthier rhythm and discover lifestyle habits that will help you address underlying factors and set the foundation for discovering your natural beauty.

There is communication between the gut microbiota and brain, and genetics and aging can impede this important relationship. The great news is that our lifestyle choices can positively improve their communication.

Stress, Aging, and Skin

There's no escaping stress. But when we let it rule our lives, problems spring up. Taming inevitable stressors in life requires creativity and focus, but the task is worth it to help our bodies' ability to restore homeostasis.

Chronic stress ages us more rapidly from the inside out, and we can see the physical and mental effects of this illness in our friends and family. Research has shown that chronic anxiety shortened telomere length in women who were middle-aged and older.[42] Telomeres are the protective caps at the end of our chromosomes, and when they shorten, it weakens their structural integrity, which means cells will age faster.

The good news is that managing stress smartly can help block this accelerated aging effect. Research suggests that mindfulness meditation[43] can lead to increased telomerase activity, and a regular meditation practice may help slow the epigenetic clock,[44] especially when practiced long term. These positive effects may cross over to the skin. Research also suggests that stress management can have a beneficial effect on skin barrier recovery before and after physical injury so that our skin looks more vibrant.[45]

In addition to accelerating aging and contributing to the development of skin conditions, being chronically stressed can make us moody. When we experience ongoing stress, our adrenal hormone cortisol increases, and our neurotransmitters serotonin and dopamine drop. These chemical messengers furthermore help with our sleep, energy, sex drive, appetite, and mood; when they're out of sync, we don't feel like our best selves.

When we're frazzled, sad, or anxious, it's harder to connect with others socially, which can make us feel lonely. This throws us into a vicious cycle of pulling back from the very things that help us feel happier and more connected—socializing with friends, exercising, getting outdoors, eating healthfully, and taking time for soothing self-care. To stop this insidious process, we will look at the root causes to understand what creates the disconnect and discover how to restore harmony. This ties back to becoming attuned to the environment once again. Studies have indicated that in general, spending time in nature helps alleviate stress, increase self-esteem, reduce anxiety, and improve mood.[46]

Education is a powerful tool. When we understand our chemical messengers and the roles that genetics, our behavior, and our environment play, we can make necessary shifts for our mental and emotional well-being. We all have had stressful and traumatic moments in our lives, certainly some of us more than others. Whether you're currently going through a stressful time, recovering from a past traumatic event, or simply wanting to improve your stress response, understanding how stress and our microbiota impact our biochemistry is an important step toward healing. And ultimately, this knowledge base will help you follow the Natural Beauty Reset program in part II.

CHAPTER 4

TIME TO RESTORE

Many of us have been there: staring at the ceiling, watching the clock, going through the to-do list in our head, and knowing we have to sleep. But try as we may, we just can't! Lack of sleep is a surefire way to feel and look tired, and it plagues many of us. In fact, I've lost count of the number of patients who have struggled with sleepless nights such as this.

Take Susan, a forty-two-year-old flight attendant who came to see me because she tossed and turned every night, and then struggled to get through her day with multiple cups of coffee, leaving her irritable and wired yet still tired.

High-quality sleep and breathing are essential for humans not only to survive but to thrive as well. However, most of us don't get the right balance of these, and it puts stress on our bodies. The good news

is being aware of these issues and making adjustments in our lifestyle can significantly improve how we sleep and breathe, thereby supporting a natural beauty reset.

Sleep deprivation can have immediate unwanted effects from making us feel cranky, angry, or sad to increasing our likelihood of making mistakes. Lack of sleep can also contribute to the risk of serious ailments such as diabetes, certain types of cancer (such as breast and ovarian), heart disease, and stroke. What's more, not snoozing enough has been linked to changes in the hormones leptin and ghrelin, which can lead to overeating and potentially to weight gain.

As if the aforementioned reasons weren't enough incentive to get more shut-eye, lack of sleep can cause puffiness and dark circles under the eyes, as well as dull skin.

Elevated levels of the stress hormone cortisol can cause a breakdown in collagen over time, which leads to accelerated fine lines and wrinkles. As a result of lack of sleep, our bodies cannot produce an adequate amount of growth hormone, which helps maintain skin thickness, muscle mass, and bone strength.

Fortunately, following a natural beauty reset can help restore balance. And just as Susan discovered after coming to see me, even though sleeping soundly seemed out of reach, it can be experienced again.

Helping women get back to a good night's rest is one of the most rewarding accomplishments I like to help my patients achieve. When we get a deep sleep and wake feeling refreshed, everything else is easier—eating healthier, exercising regularly, making informed choices, enjoying sex, and feeling more joyful with a sense of peace. This all leads to a healthier glow!

One way to get back to sleeping soundly is by developing body awareness. Being aware of your body's messages is one of the best ways we can restore our natural rhythms. Our bodies are designed with certain feedback mechanisms to let us know we need to adjust. While we breathe and sleep without having to think about it, we shouldn't ignore the feedback signals. I'll explain why and help you determine if you are optimizing them. But first, let's cover some physiology basics so you understand how and why lifestyle shifts are critical for a good night's sleep.

Our circadian rhythm is our internal biological clock, which is key for restorative beauty sleep. It is controlled by an area in the hypothalamus of the brain called the suprachiasmatic nucleus (SCN), which senses light and dark. When the optic nerve in our eyes senses light, the SCN causes the release of certain hormones such as cortisol that help us wake up, and with darkness, the SCN sends signals to the pineal gland to release melatonin. Changes in seasons affect our melatonin as well as serotonin production, which can impact our sleep and, in turn, our mood and cognition.[47]

While melatonin is the main hormone typically thought of when it comes to sleep, simply popping a melatonin supplement is not always going to help you catch your z's. For example, adenosine, a neurochemical that acts as a sleep signal, and caffeine, which helps us stay alert by blocking adenosine's receptors, also play a role in quality slumber.

In general, avoid caffeine at least six hours before bedtime. That's the typical amount of time it takes us to clear caffeine from our bodies, though everyone's different. If you're sensitive to caffeine like I am, cut out caffeine or limit your consumption to the morning.

Alcohol consumption also is known to interfere with our sleep. While alcohol can make us feel drowsy, it disrupts our natural sleep patterns, decreasing REM (deep) sleep and contributing to sleep apnea, a common disorder that causes abnormal breathing and temporary pauses in breathing during sleep. At the very least, avoid alcohol four hours before bedtime to help ensure a good night's sleep.

For many of my patients, removing alcohol from their evening routines has helped reduce night sweats, hot flashes, and difficulty sleeping. With that in mind, you may want to try cutting out alcohol for one to two weeks and notice how your sleep quality changes, or limit alcohol consumption to weekends rather than every night. If you're like many of my patients, you may find that you're healthier and happier.

Another lesser-discussed hormone released during sleep is vasopressin, which triggers our bodies to store water and not be thirsty at night. But if we don't get enough deep sleep, then vasopressin doesn't do its job and an overnight urge to urinate or hydrate happens. Lack of vasopressin further disrupts our sleep and may contribute to dehydration.[48] Alcohol and caffeine consumption also suppresses the release of vasopressin, which is another reason these are best avoided before bedtime.

Out of Circadian Sync

While artificial light has illuminated our living spaces when it's dark out, it has caused circadian desynchrony, taking an unfortunate toll on our bodies and brains.[49] Among its downsides, light at night negatively affects mood[50] and eating habits, increasing the risk for weight gain.[51] It's no wonder our bodies have

gotten unhealthier inside and out, with the advent of artificial light.

Compared to red light, blue light is more stimulating to our system. Red light sources include the sun and incandescent light bulbs, whereas blue light comes from electronic devices. Wisely, the sun transmits more blue light during the day than at sunset. However, nighttime tech routines undermine this natural cycle—and our sleep takes a hit in turn.

One step you can take to reduce exposure to sleep-interfering blue light is to avoid or limit use of devices such as cell phones, laptops, computers, e-readers, and TVs at least two hours before bedtime. If giving up your electronic devices before bed is not an option, dim the lighting on the devices and get blue-light-blocking devices, such as amber-lensed glasses.[52] Studies have shown that wearing these two hours before bedtime for one week improved sleep in people with insomnia. Another tip is to dim and even change the lighting in your bedroom and other rooms where you are spending time before bed from blue light (fluorescent and LED) to yellow or orange.

Besides light, a major contributor of circadian desynchrony is temperature. Our body temperature drops at night.[53] We are more likely to fall asleep when our body temperature is dropping rather than rising. For that reason, if you have difficulty sleeping or to improve your night's sleep, first make sure your bedroom thermostat is lower at night than during the day, ideally around 65 degrees Fahrenheit.[54] If that doesn't help, try taking a warm bath before bedtime. When you get out of the warm bath, the cooler air temperature will cause a drop in your body temperature, signaling that it's time for sleep. Keep in mind that the temperature change should be mild because if you try to drop the temperature in the room or your body too quickly, your body may experience that as stress and it will interfere with sleep.

Humidity levels may also play a role in sleep. Ideally, the humidity level in your bedroom ought to be 40 to 60 percent. So if you live in a place where it's fairly humid, you're likely within that range. But if you live in a drier climate, then you may want to consider putting a humidifier in your bedroom to help aid sleep.

In addition to our environment, breathing plays an instrumental role in biological harmony. We breathe involuntarily, but that doesn't mean we're performing this action optimally. Breathing is much more than just an oxygen and carbon dioxide exchange. The way we breathe can impact our heart rate, mood, sexual arousal, and digestion. While sleeping, many of us breathe through our mouths, snore, or struggle with sleep apnea—all of which impede our sleep.

Deep breathing offers established health benefits.[55] Our parasympathetic nervous system aids with rest and digestion, while the sympathetic nervous system helps us with fight-or-flight. There are many parasympathetic system nerves in the lower lobes of our lungs, which is part of the reason taking deep breaths helps us feel calm. A prolonged exhale triggers even more activity and feelings of relaxation—slowing our heart rate and making us feel more at ease.

Many of the sympathetic nerves are located at the tops of our lungs, so when we take a lot of short breaths, it can trigger the fight-or-flight response. While the sympathetic dominant state prepares our body for danger and can help us survive an emergency, we're only designed to stay in that state for short periods of time. So it's essential to find balance with our breathing.

Here is a simple breathwork exercise to help you reconnect, rebalance, and prepare your body for sleep:

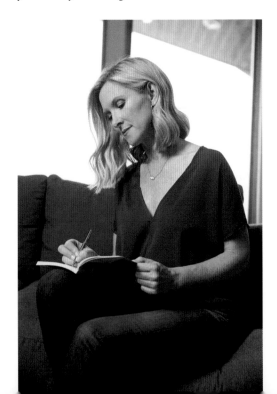

While keeping your mouth closed, inhale slowly and deeply through your nose for a count of five, focusing on expanding your belly as you breathe in. Then exhale through your nose for a count of five and bring your belly back in toward your spine. Repeat this five-count inhale and five-count exhale for at least two minutes. When you notice your body relaxing and your mind quieting, you can return to normal breathing. Or if you're doing this in bed, you can continue this breathing until you fall asleep.

When and how you move your body plays a significant role in sleep and restoration. While beneficial in the morning, vigorous exercise too close to bedtime (within ninety minutes) may impede your ability to unwind in time to maintain a healthy sleep schedule. Therefore, I recommend reserving more strenuous exercises for early in the day and more relaxing movement toward the late afternoon and evening.

Equally important is forming a sleep ritual that works for your unique chemistry. Sleep is sacred time, so you'll want to build a routine that soothes the senses to prepare your mind and body for a restorative night's sleep. Lighting a candle, listening to calming music, taking a relaxing bath with mineral salts and lavender or rose essential oils, sipping on chamomile tea, taking deep cleansing breaths, and writing in a gratitude journal are some ways you can shift your mood and mindset.

I give recommendations for sleep rituals in part II for each season, and here are some year-round tips to set you up for a restorative night's sleep.

YEAR-ROUND SLEEP TIPS

❄ Cut caffeine by 2 PM. Caffeine has a half-life of eight to ten hours, so stop drinking caffeine by the early afternoon.

❄ Limit (or avoid) your evening intake of alcohol. Booze prevents deeper stages of sleep, so stop drinking it at least four hours before bed.

❄ Exercise regularly but not too much. Exercising in the morning or afternoon is the best way to improve overall sleep quality.

❄ Trim your tech habit. Blue light keeps us awake, so reduce electronic exposure before bedtime.

❄ Turn down the sounds. Turn off the television and shift to a more quiet atmosphere. If you need some sound to help you sleep, white noise is fine.

❄ Keep your room chilly. Adjust the temperature in the room to 65 to 75 degrees Fahrenheit.

❄ Create a comfy space. The pillows and mattresses matter.

❄ Turn to soothing scents. Lavender is helpful.

❄ Try tracking your sleep with a wearable device. Aim for five ninety-minute cycles, which comes out to seven and a

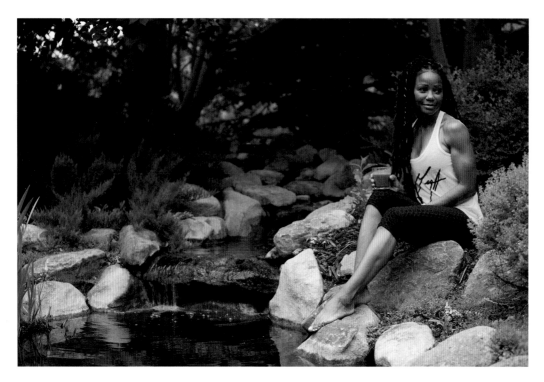

half hours. This is a great place to start, and then you can customize your sleep cycle as you see fit.

❖ Wake up with sunlight. When sunlight hits the optic nerve in the morning hours, it stops melatonin production and wakes you up. Aim for fifteen minutes of sun exposure when you rise.

If you still need help, consider supplementation. You can find melatonin supplements in a range of dosages and forms, but the most common is 0.3 to 5.0 mg in a sublingual pill or swallowable capsule. When I recommend melatonin to my patients, I tell them to take it forty-five to sixty minutes before bedtime. While melatonin supplements are generally safe to take and side effects are rare, some people may experience symptoms such as nightmares, headaches, nausea, and agitation. If you develop symptoms or your sleep does not improve, talk with your doctor. Remember that there is more than low melatonin that can cause you to have sleepless nights, so melatonin supplementation isn't for everyone.

You can find other opportunities to restore and reset throughout your day. Taking time to close your eyes, do deep belly breathing, and clear your mind of negative thoughts can do wonders to decrease stress hormones and boost your feel-good neurotransmitters. You deserve this time to yourself!

CHAPTER 5

FOOD, HABITS, AND SEASONAL CHANGES

"Let food be thy medicine and let medicine be thy food" is a quote attributed to Hippocrates, and food is certainly a key part of the Natural Beauty Reset program. Our food supply changes with seasons, as do our hormones and habits. They're all beautifully interconnected.

Sunlight Exposure and Hormones

As seasons change, so does the amount of time we are exposed to sunlight. In autumn and winter, for instance, the days are shorter than those in the summertime, which means less sun exposure. Reduced sunlight influences our behaviors and our

food cravings, and the underlying reason has to do with our chemical messengers.

The changes in sunlight exposure align with those of our hormones. I mentioned some of these shifts in earlier chapters, but here's a quick refresher: research suggests that our cortisol levels are typically higher in fall and winter compared to spring and summer.[56] Cortisol levels may affect factors such as mood, appetite, and weight, so these seasonal changes may make us prone to be drawn to comfort foods to ease our stress.

Because leptin is typically higher in the winter and ghrelin is lower, our appetites may be lower in the winter.[57] As days get shorter and longer, melatonin production fluctuates as well. With shorter daylight hours in winter, we have greater melatonin production compared to summer. And with those fluctuations come changes in other hormones, such as sex and thyroid hormones, triggering alterations in our energy and desire.[58]

Spring's reputation for being a time of high fertility is well founded. Estrogen levels in women tend to rise in spring,[59] as do sperm counts[60] in men. These effects increase our chances of conception.

I share this insight on seasonal hormonal shifts to illustrate how they can actually work in our favor if we manage stress, improve sleep, and balance hormones, making adjustments with the seasons. Knowing about these changes can help us understand why at certain times we may tend to put on weight, feel unmotivated, or experience certain food cravings. For optimal health and natural beauty, it's essential to shift our habits according to the seasons to restore hormonal harmony. I will explain exactly how to do that in part II, but for now let's look at seasonal changes that play a role in our food and nutrient supplies.

Sunlight Exposure and Food

The seasonal changes also influence our nutritional status. Because sun exposure is the primary driver of natural vitamin D production in the body, our levels tend to dip in the wintertime. Meanwhile, we receive other vitamins as well as minerals from plants, which are not immune to the effects of seasonal changes, either.

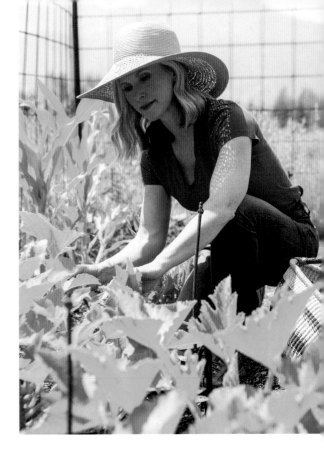

Namely, shifts in day length can affect how and which types of produce grow well. For example, hardier plants like kale flourish in the fall and springtime months, when temperatures tend to be cool. Even in places like California and Arizona, which some people may describe as seasonless, various types of produce grow best at certain times of the year because of changes in the sun's location and the duration of sunlight hours.

Educating ourselves about seasonal eating wasn't always necessary—it was simply a part of life. That is, humans used to grow and raise their own food out of necessity, and they had no choice but to eat according to the seasons. But now, many of us can get any food from anywhere at just about any time of day, month, or year.

Think of it like this: We may look up a salad recipe that calls for broccoli as its main green. It happens to be spring when we have this hankering. So we head to the grocery store and pick up a head of broccoli without another thought. Here's the thing: the nutritional profile of that broccoli has almost double the levels of vitamin C when you enjoy it during its peak freshness—that is, during late fall compared to spring.[61] The researchers who observed this intended to determine the difference between conventionally grown versus organic produce, but, in the end, they found the growing season had the biggest effect on the level of vitamin C in broccoli! In buying produce that's out of season, we're ultimately sacrificing nutritional value and taste—the latter of which you'll know well when you've had produce in season.

Buying produce in season isn't exactly the norm, so it's no surprise that our average levels of nutrients like folate are lower during winter and spring, when foods rich in folate, like dark-green leafy vegetables, are less abundant.[62] Folate plays a role in serotonin production and adrenal function, and a deficiency has been linked to depression and fatigue.

Already, many Americans are at risk for nutrient deficiencies due to following the standard American diet. This eating pattern is low in fruits and veggies, and

high in processed foods replete with added sugar, sodium, and saturated fat that can wreak havoc on hormonal harmony as well as our holistic health. Coupled with eating produce out of season, these unfortunately common eating habits can make for an imbalanced body.

While a big focus in this chapter is on seasonal changes of plants, meat eaters can benefit from understanding the inner workings and benefits of seasonal eating, too. That's because animals such as chickens and cows also consume plants.

Food-Growing Practices and Gut Health

Understanding when our food is grown or prepared is important, but so is knowing where it came from and how it came about.

Plant-based foods like fruits and veggies get their nutrients from the soil in which they are grown. The truth is, popular farming practices use nutrient-depleted soil, which may prevent plant foods from reaching their full nutritional potential. Unfortunately, even the healthiest of foods (such as green, leafy veggies) can be deficient in their natural nutrients.

In addition to the bounty of vitamins and minerals present in quality soil, there is an interesting parallel between soil quality and our microbiome. The soil and the human gut contain about the same number of active microorganisms, and yet the average human gut microbiome is only

10 percent as diverse as that of soil. What's going on? You may be able to guess. The realities of modern life have messed with human health. Indeed, the diversity of human gut bacteria decreased significantly as we transitioned from a hunter-gatherer to an urbanized society.[63]

In short, understanding the origin and quality of our food, and considering whether it is plant-based fare or meat, is crucial to ensuring we're filling our plates in a way that not only nourishes our bodies to the maximum benefit, but also enables hormonal harmony. Plus, acknowledging and valuing the origin of our food, such as when you support local farmers at the market, can benefit our communities and may help fatten our wallets by helping us save money. (Yes, buying in-season produce tends to be less expensive than produce that is out of season!)[64]

Food Preservatives and Environmental Impact

In addition to the way food is grown, consider how it may be transported to the grocery store. Many produce suppliers use post-harvest treatments[65] such as heat, irradiation, and adding edible coatings[66] to reduce spoilage and slow ripening during transport. This makes for long-lasting produce that manufacturers can sell en masse, but this approach prevents you from maximizing the perks of such produce. Here's why: produce is often harvested before it's

fully ripe, which means it has less time to mature at its source for full nourishment. When you eat seasonally and locally grown produce, you can help minimize or avoid these issues.

Not to be overlooked are the environmental effects these food-manufacturing practices can pose. Specifically, greenhouses growing out-of-season produce require more energy and therefore expand their carbon footprint.[67]

Overall, it can be helpful to understand how our modern lifestyle has contributed to some of the underlying issues of nutritional deficiencies, microbiome disturbances, and hormonal imbalances. The good news is that we can strike a balance between getting reattuned to nature and enjoying the luxuries of this day and age while still nourishing our bodies optimally. I will discuss how to do just that in part II.

Whole Versus Processed Food

Overall, healthy eating can be intuitive, and yet we often overcomplicate it. We can become confused by all of the various diets we have to choose from today. Aligning with our ideal food choices doesn't have to be complicated, though. Simply put, the closer our food is to nature (meaning it's fresh, local, and seasonal), the higher its nutritional content. Meanwhile, the more processed our food is, the less nourishment it provides.

Why do we want to take this approach to eating for natural beauty? Let's start with the fact that fresh, local, and seasonal produce is rich in nutrients like antioxidants that help protect us against harmful, disease-promoting oxidative damage. Oxidative damage also impacts our hormones, as free radicals can interfere with pituitary hormones.[68] We need certain nutrients from food for hormonal balance.

But, if nature is so healing, then why do we crave processed foods?

I grew up in the South (where fried Coca-Cola is actually a thing) and understand the desires we have for comfort foods. I remember my great-aunt Betty saying about her recipe for broccoli, "After I steam it, I add just a wee bit of sugar because everything is better with just a little bit of sugar!" And food-packaging companies seem to agree with Aunt Betty because they seemingly add sugar to all kinds of foods. From crackers and bread to spreads and salad dressings, sugar is lurking everywhere, and not always in plain sight.

Health-wise, excess sugar intake is costly. It has been linked to obesity, diabetes, certain types of cancer, and suppressed immune system activity. Regular sugar consumption also negatively impacts many of our hormones, including cortisol, thyroid (T3 and T4), and insulin. In turn, our energy, metabolism, mood, and sleep quality take a hit. Plus, the effects often show up on our skin as acne and accelerated signs of aging.

Sugar is addictive like a drug, and we easily can get caught in a vicious cycle with our hormones and emotional food choices.[69] When we crave comfort food and sweets, our hormones are often out of balance. When we crave ice cream and chocolate chip cookies, our bodies are actually starving for hormonal harmony!

I've seen hundreds of patients struggle with sugar, and I have successfully helped them get to the root of the issue, return to intuitive eating, restore their health, and reset their hormones to optimal levels. For example, Katherine was a thirty-seven-year-old mother of three who came to see me with irregular cycles and PMS. As a single mother, she was trying to do it all—raise her children and manage a work-life balance. And she had a secret: she used peanut M&M's as her stress management. An integral part of her treatment plan was helping wean her off high-sugar foods and onto a more balanced nutritional meal plan. After a week of my reset program, Katherine started noticing her cravings subside, and she was able to intuitively make healthier eating choices. She also learned some more effective stress-management techniques.

There's no shame here! We all have cravings, and it's okay if you want to treat yourself now and then. The point is that we are striving for balance, and part of that balance is managing being human. We live in a time when sugary and processed foods are replete, and for many of us they are nostalgic. If you want to indulge occasionally, do it mindfully.

Because elevated blood sugar, oxidative damage, gut microbiome imbalances, and nutritional deficiencies are core root causes that you can address through your lifestyle, you'll want to start with giving your body a break from the foods that trigger internal inflammation, like sugar and alcohol. Instead, restore the body with nourishing foods. This will help your hormonal harmony as your body will have the nutrients and environment needed to make and metabolize hormones.

Adjusting Eating as We Age

The other factor that influences nourishment from food stems from our gut. We could eat the healthiest foods on the planet, but if our digestion and absorption is malfunctioning, we will not get the nutrients from food that we deserve.

To further complicate the issue, these problems worsen with age. For one, hydrochloric acid levels, which aid in our digestion, decrease as we age, so the body's ability to digest and absorb nutrients from our food the same way we used to declines. This means our requirements for macronutrients and micronutrients—those essential nutrients we get from food—change. We're not growing as we did in our youth, but we still need these nutrients to support skin repair and help prevent oxidative damage. Because of these changes, we may experience more delayed wound healing and less vibrant-looking skin, among other effects.

If you weren't aware of the benefits of seasonal eating, are concerned about poor gut health, or simply believe you've been doing your body a disservice in the nutrition department, you may feel discouraged. But don't worry. You aren't alone. In part II, I'll show you how to optimize your digestion and assimilation as well as your nutritional status and hormonal balance for graceful aging and natural beauty!

CHAPTER 6

TOO
TOXIC

We are commonly exposed to toxins via our personal-care products, food, water, home environments, hobby supplies, and work environments. The idea is to be aware of these exposures so we can be empowered with solutions to reduce our exposure to toxins and keep hormones balanced for natural beauty and vibrant health.

As the human population has grown and technology has advanced, environmental exposure to toxins has unfortunately increased. In addition to the new toxic chemicals product manufacturers are creating at this very moment, many exist already in our air, water, food sources, and personal-care products. These toxins include lead, mercury, arsenic, bisphenol-A (BPA), and phthalates. As mentioned, EDC exposures can

trigger hormonal imbalances, which is the very thing we're trying to avoid when doing a natural beauty reset.

While the skin as well as the liver, kidney, and lymphatic and digestive systems naturally eliminate harmful invaders from the body, sometimes the influx of toxins is too great a burden for the body to bear. And some toxins, such as lead and mercury, store within the body more readily than others. When these levels increase in our bodies, we can become acutely and chronically sick, develop hormonal imbalances, and experience accelerated aging.

One of the biggest accelerators in premature aging is due to oxidative damage. This process occurs internally from exposure to toxins and unhealthy lifestyle choices such as eating processed foods and too much sugar. Oxidative damage can lead to DNA telomere shortening and genetic alterations, thereby accelerating signs of aging. Beyond aging, oxidative damage plays a role in the development of significant health challenges such as cancer, diabetes, and Alzheimer's disease.

In the skin, free radicals damage collagen, resulting in sagging, dullness, and uneven tone. External exposure to pollutants in the air and skincare products, as well as excess sun exposure, trigger oxidative damage. This, in turn, accelerates the aforementioned signs of premature aging.

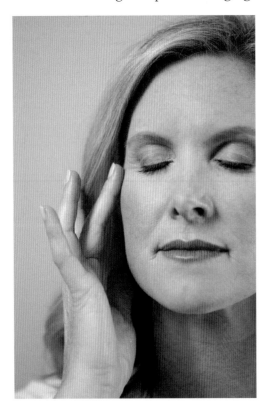

Oxidative damage already happens naturally with age. In the skin specifically, levels of antioxidants—which help combat oxidative damage—decline as the years pass. This makes healthy diet and lifestyle changes even more important. Eating foods high in antioxidants (many of which you'll find inspiration for in the recipes section) is one way to help protect the body, including the skin, against the harmful effects of this process.

Toxins in Skincare

Think about all of the lipsticks, mascaras, eyeshadows, foundations, sunscreens, masks, cleansers, creams, and lotions in bathroom drawers and cabinets (and don't forget the ones in your purse!). It adds up, right? One study suggests the average woman owns forty makeup products.[70] And according to the Environmental Working Group, women use an average of twelve personal-care products each day, potentially exposing them to 168 unique ingredients.[71]

Even if you like your thorough skincare routine, be mindful that what you put on your skin is absorbed, to a certain extent, into your body and may elevate the level of toxins you're already exposed to each day. Ingredients found in popular skincare products have been shown to cause endocrine-disrupting effects, and some are even carcinogenic—two things no one wants to deal with.

Unfortunately, the FDA in the United States does not require safety testing of skincare ingredients and has only banned 11 ingredients for use in personal-care products.[72] The European Union, on the other hand, has banned over 1,300 ingredients in personal-care products because of their connection to genetic mutation, reproductive concerns, and cancer. Especially if you live in the United States, it's up to you to take a closer look at what you're putting on your body.

Here are three examples of potentially toxic ingredients in skincare products that may disrupt hormones:

1. Parabens: We know from research that parabens are absorbed through the skin and can be taken up and stored in our body's tissues. Used in many personal-care products as preservatives, parabens have been detected in breast tumor tissue and are known to have estrogen-mimicking effects. One study found a correlation between lower circulating thyroid hormone levels in adults who had higher paraben levels in their urine—with the strongest and most consistent associations among females.[73] To identify parabens on skincare labels, look for *propylparaben*, *benzylparaben*, *methylparaben*, or *butylparaben*.

2. Fragrance: We like to smell good, and product manufacturers know that. Fragrance is not a single ingredient, even though it is listed that way, and can contain a number of EDCs, such as diethyl phthalate (DEP).

Researchers who published their findings in *Environmental Health Perspectives* found metabolites of DEP and other phthalates in more than 75 percent of the 2,540 samples collected from participants of the National Health and Nutrition Examination Survey.[74] In another report published in the *International Journal of Hygiene and Environmental Health*, researchers detected eleven phthalate metabolites in more than 90 percent of Canadians surveyed in the Canadian Health Measures Survey from 2007 to 2009.[75] These statistics suggest widespread exposure and absorption of phthalates in the United States and Canada.

3. Oxybenzone (benzophenone): Benzophenone-type UV filters are a common active ingredient in chemical sun protection products such as sunscreen and lip balms, and research suggests these have hormone-disrupting effects. Oxybenzone isn't the only sunscreen ingredient linked with hormone-disrupting effects—it's best to steer clear of octinoxate and homosalate, too. A clinical trial published in the *Journal of the American Medical Association* found all six active ingredients in sunscreens that were tested (avobenzone, oxybenzone, octocrylene, homosalate, octisalate, and octinoxate) were systemically absorbed,

and blood levels surpassed the FDA's threshold.[76] While these chemical sunscreen ingredients are still recommended, I think it's safer to swap to mineral-based sunscreens.

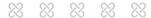

Instead of synthetic fragrance, choose pure essential oils such as ylang-ylang and bergamot. Replace synthetic toxic preservatives with natural ingredients, including rosemary extract and citric acid, that can work wonderfully as part of a natural preservative system. And when you're stepping out into the sun, you can protect your skin with a zinc oxide–based mineral, or physical sunscreens in lieu of chemical products.

Let's face it. Avoiding all EDC exposure is impossible. But knowing the possible risks, why would we want to worsen the problem by using affected personal-care products when you have alternative choices? I will cover seasonal skincare recommendations that highlight natural ingredients in part II, but for now let's turn to what toxins you may be putting *in* your body.

Toxins in Food and Drinks

Ideally, the food we eat should nourish our bodies. But unfortunately, our food can be a source of toxin exposure if we don't choose wisely. Here are some of the most common toxins in food, food storage, and food preparation:

- Lead and pesticides: There can be heavy metals in our air, water, and soil that can end up in our food supply. Lead is one example.[77] Although manufacturers of paint and gasoline are no longer permitted to use this naturally occurring element in their products, it still exists in soil.[78] That means lead can end up in grains, fruits, and vegetables, and meat eaters have additional exposure because the animals we eat consume this produce. Pesticides linked to endocrine-disrupting effects as well as cancer are sprayed on produce grown today, and genetically modified foods bring an additional layer of complexity with long-term safety concerns for us and the planet.

- PCBs and mercury: Fish, especially those higher up on the food chain—the large ones such as swordfish and king mackerel, which eat smaller fish—as well as shellfish, tend to bioaccumulate toxic chemicals that have been linked to serious health concerns, including cancer.[79] These chemicals include polychlorinated biphenyls (PCBs)[80] and mercury.[81]

- BPA: Beyond the food itself, storage has the potential to create additional toxic exposures. For example, BPA is a chemical found in plastic food packaging and food storage containers, as well as in the lining of cans, and is known to leach into the food and drinks that it comes in contact with.[82] BPA exposure has been linked to breast cancer,[83] pregnancy complications with the developing fetus, type 2 diabetes,[84] obesity, PCOS,[85] infertility,[86] and altered thyroid hormone production. You can reduce your exposure to BPA and similar toxic chemicals by buying fresh whole foods rather than processed fare, and by using fabric bags, glass, ceramic, and stainless-steel containers for food and drink storage.

❄ Oxidized oils and PAHs: Cooking methods also have the potential to make our food toxic to our health. Fats and oils cooked at high temperature, such as when frying, easily become oxidized, which increases our free radical exposure. To avoid these concerns, you can focus on cooking your food at lower temperatures by steaming and baking. When you do use oils, use those that are more stable at higher temperatures such as coconut and avocado oils. If you enjoy grilling your food, know that barbecued meats and other overcooked meats release polycyclic aromatic hydrocarbons (PAHs), which have been linked to cancer.[87]

❄ HFCS and sugar: High-fructose corn syrup (HFCS) and sugar can be toxic to our bodies if consumed in excess. When we overdo it with sugar consumption, we may be at higher risk for breast cancer,[88] type 2 diabetes,[89] insulin resistance,[90] colon cancer,[91]

and cardiovascular disease.[92] We can reduce our risk by limiting sugar intake, and when we do consume sweets, focusing on natural forms such as honey, maple syrup, and stevia is best. Don't forget to watch out for hidden sources of the sweet stuff such as in sports drinks, bottled fruit juices, condiments, sauces, and dressings.

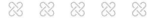

While some toxins in the environment are unavoidable, you can shift your eating habits to significantly reduce your exposures. Additionally, you can eat to enhance your detoxification pathways to help support your body function as it was designed—to eliminate toxic foreign substances. And this is precisely the kind of eating plan you'll find in part II.

Toxins in the Home and Workplace

Hobbies help us relax and unwind, so we sometimes overlook them as a possible toxin exposure. If you have hobbies such as painting, jewelry making, furniture restoration, sculpting, or photography, look at the ingredient labels (or online) and avoid those with heavy metals such as arsenic and lead and other toxic ingredients. And be sure to do these in well-ventilated areas.

Home is a place where we can rest, rebalance, and restore, so the last thing you want to do is bring toxins into this haven. Unfortunately, though, toxins are in common household products, including those we use to clean our bathrooms and clothing, as well as those we use to prevent pests from invading.

The good news is we can choose nontoxic products that will still keep our homes safe and clean, while allowing us to stay healthy and in hormonal harmony. These products also tend to be more environmentally friendly than their toxic counterparts! Believe it or not, furniture, rugs, and carpeting are major contributors of indoor air pollution, so it's best to choose natural fibers and solid wood furnishings to avoid the off-gassing of volatile organic compounds (VOCs). You may want to consider an air purifier for your home, particularly in areas where you spend a lot of time such as in your bedroom.

Even though it is technically natural, mold is also a toxin. Mold exists to break things down, which is actually a good thing for nature, but we don't want mold in our homes and workplaces. If you notice a water leak, repair it quickly and thoroughly to avoid mold exposure, and make sure moist areas such as bathrooms are well ventilated. If you suspect you have mold, have your home tested and handled by a mold remediation professional.

While we have less control over public workplaces, we can certainly help make a change. After all, the toxins that affect you also impact your colleagues. Consider your air supply, too. Ask questions such as how often the furnaces are cleaned and if the business can switch to nontoxic cleaning products. Ask if you can bring in a small personal air purification unit for your workspace.

TIPS TO REDUCE TOXIN EXPOSURES

Personal-care products:

* Avoid toxic ingredients. See a list of twenty personal-care product ingredients to avoid in chapter 10 in the spring skincare cleanup. You can find more about these ingredients in my book *Clean Skin from Within* and others at www.ewg.org/skindeep.

* Swap out toxic ingredients for natural ones such as organic essential oils; aloe vera; green, black, and white teas; rosemary extract; sunflower seed oil; apricot kernel oil; almond oil; jojoba oil; resveratrol; vitamin E; CoQ10; and turmeric. You can find all of these in The Spa Dr.'s Daily Essentials skincare.

* Choose skincare lines made with organic, nongenetically modified (non-GM), and wild-crafted ingredients. See the resources section at the back of this book for recommendations.

* In addition to skincare and makeup, replace your deodorant, shampoo, conditioner, and other personal-care products that have toxic ingredients with nontoxic, natural alternatives.

Don't forget that unless they're organic, your feminine hygiene products contain pesticides and other potentially toxic ingredients.

Food and beverages:

Choose organic as much as possible, especially those on the Environmental Working Group's dirty dozen list, which are known to be the top fruits and vegetables with pesticide residues.[93]

Choose fresh and local over packaged and processed foods as much as possible.

When buying food stored in plastic and cans, choose BPA-free.

Store food and beverages in glass, stainless steel, and ceramic containers.

Choose wild-caught over farm-raised fish, and choose fish known to be lower in mercury and PCBs, such as those listed on the National Resources Defense Council (NRDC)'s wallet guide.[94]

If you eat meat, choose organic, grass-fed, free-range, and pasture-raised varieties.

Read your food labels to reduce your exposure to toxic chemical ingredients and excess sugar.

Drink filtered water. Reverse osmosis is my favorite type of water filter because it removes the most toxins from water, but it also removes minerals. If you use this product, consider a system that replenishes minerals, or use mineral supplements.

Replace your Teflon and other nonstick cookware with stainless steel, glass, ceramic, or cast-iron to avoid perfluorooctanoic acid and other chemicals that may be linked to cancer and other health concerns.

Home and work:

Reduce moisture by ensuring spaces like bathrooms are well ventilated to avoid mold growth, and be sure to fix water damage quickly and thoroughly.

Use nontoxic eco-friendly cleaning and laundry products.

Choose furniture and home goods made of solid wood and natural fabrics.

Select organic natural-fiber clothing (such as bamboo, cotton, and wool), when possible, and wash new clothing before wearing.

When renovating, choose low- or no-VOC paints and look for sustainable and nontoxic options.

Avoid pesticides and herbicides in and around your house, and instead look for natural, nontoxic alternatives.

Consider placing one or more air purifiers in your home or workplace. My favorites are those made by Austin Air, Blueair, and IQAir.

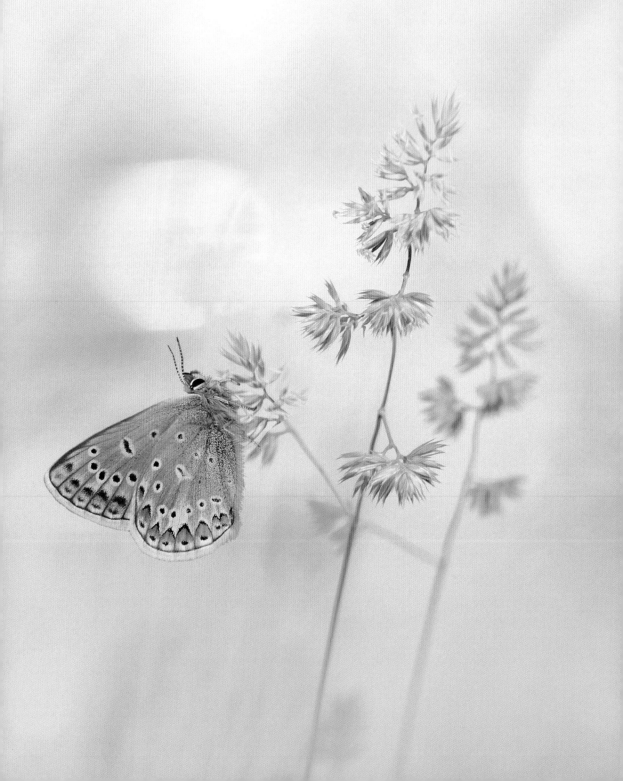

PART II

The 7-Day Natural Beauty Reset Program

This program shows you how to turn to nature and reset your lifestyle for harmonious hormones and vibrant health. You will discover how to reconnect with your body's wisdom and glow in a way you may never have thought possible.

It's clear that adopting a healthy lifestyle—including nourishing our bodies with quality food, getting regular physical activity, deploying effective stress-management techniques, and designing an informed skincare routine—impacts our bodies' aging process inside and out.[95] The point of this reset is much more than to delay early signs of aging; it's to restore your natural beauty and build resilience so you're able to age gracefully and be less likely to get sick. So it will be important to pay attention to those eating and lifestyle habits on your journey to a natural beauty reset. My plan provides the tools, resources,

and confidence you'll need to meet your goals, all the while enhancing your natural beauty, balancing your hormones, and optimizing your internal and external health.

Part II kicks off with a year-round foundational plan for food, movement, mindset, and skincare. Here, you'll find considerations and recommendations for all four categories of the program to set you up for success. Starting in chapter 8, you'll find the 7-Day Natural Beauty Reset for fall, winter, spring, and summer. These include seasonal modifications for the aforementioned categories. In chapter 12, you'll discover how to personalize your 7-Day Natural Beauty Reset program and receive tips that, when followed, will enable you to enjoy a lifetime of natural beauty. Then, gear up your taste buds. Chapter 13 includes recipes and resources mentioned throughout part II.

CHAPTER 7

FOOD, MOVEMENT, MINDSET, AND SKINCARE FOR THE SEASONS

Starting each season with a seven-day reset is an effective yet easy way to refresh your habits and start to restore harmony. It's like pressing and holding the power button on your malfunctioning smartphone to restore its full potential and bring its bright, glowing screen back to life. This process may come with some discomfort and uncertainty—going back to the phone analogy, it may feel like you're going to lose all your data—but I promise that when you hit reset, you will feel revitalized and renewed.

Expect to feel more vibrant, energetic, and productive. All the bugs will be worked out, and you won't feel glitchy, sluggish, or tired. Your friends, family, and coworkers will see a new you, and they'll be dying to figure out your secret. Little will they realize you're the same person they've known all along; you're just revitalized, thanks to that reset.

Before we dive into the specifics for each season, let's touch on some of the basics for year-round food, movement, mindset, and skincare.

Food Basics for All Seasons

If you've ever tasted berries from the vine, apples from your local orchard, or fresh herbs from the garden, you know the difference eating foods that are in season can make. The flavor is 180 degrees different from eating packaged produce from the refrigerated section of your local grocery store. Not to mention, the closer we get to consuming our foods at their source, the more flavor and nutritional content they have.

Eating seasonally is a game changer. Once you get used to this way of eating, you won't want to go back.

To get started, look for a local source of produce such as at a corner kiosk, farmers market, or CSA (community-supported agriculture) programs. That will help ensure you are eating in-season produce for your region. I also encourage you to consider starting your own garden, even if it's a window garden with some fresh herbs. This saves you money and supports businesses in your community. Who knows, you may even make some new friends that mirror your lifestyle.

If sourcing local produce is out of reach, try to find which of your local grocery stores has the freshest produce and largest selection of organic options. Alternatively, though less ideally, you may order certain foods online.

Some foods grow year-round, whereas others grow during a specific season or two. Some produce may grow during more than one season, so this is merely a guide to help you connect with the cycles and rhythms of nature. You also want to rely upon your intuition.

The Foundation: Planting the Seeds

Having a healthy foundation with food will help you focus on foods rich in antioxidants, collagen-boosting nutrients, and skin-loving fatty acids, all of which support hormonal balance and overall radiance. The foundational eating in this section

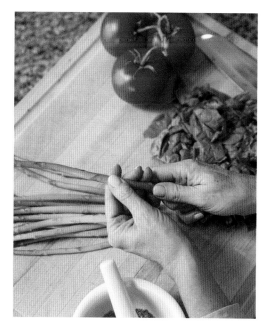

includes food groups and their portions so you can apply these principles throughout the year while making adjustments to eat foods that are harvested and readily available for each season.

FOUNDATIONAL EATING

The recommendations for serving size below are general, but everyone's needs are different. I'm not a fan of prolonged caloric restriction because I've seen it trigger eating disorders and cause bone loss and nutritional deficiencies.[96] For that reason, in this chapter you'll see minimum, not maximum, serving sizes. If you are looking for a weight loss program or want individualized nutritional guidance, I suggest working with a naturopathic physician or functional medicine doctor.

- Vegetables: Four or more servings of a variety of vegetables daily. A general serving size is 1 cup uncooked. (Tip: to get in four servings, aim for one serving of vegetables with breakfast and lunch and two with dinner.) Everyone knows they're supposed to eat more vegetables, but the key to attaining natural beauty is eating a variety of vegetables that are in season. Vegetables provide fiber, and increasing our fiber intake helps keep blood sugar levels balanced. Eating a variety of produce helps support a healthy gut microbiome. All of this helps with hormonal harmony, and when you incorporate cruciferous veggies, including broccoli, kale, cauliflower, and brussels sprouts, your estrogen metabolism benefits.

- Fruit: One or more servings daily. A general serving size is 1 cup. With fruit, we want to focus on those that are nutrient dense. Avocados and olives are actually fruits, not vegetables, and they're known to be rich in monounsaturated fats and antioxidants. Other fruits like berries, apples, cherries, and pears are also rich in antioxidants and are great when in season.

- Nuts and seeds: At least two servings daily (two or more if you're vegetarian). A general serving size is about ¼ cup nuts and seeds or 2 tablespoons of nut butter. Nuts and seeds are small but mighty. They provide healthy fats, protein, and micronutrients that we need for healthy hormones and to feel satiated. Enjoy them as a snack or as an addition to your meals.

- Clean protein: At least two servings per day of animal (meat, fish, dairy, eggs) or plant (legumes such as beans and peas) proteins, or both. A general serving size is 3 ounces of meat or fish, two eggs, 1 cup dairy, and ¾ cup legumes. If you're an omnivore, ideally, you will consume both legumes and animal protein, but you can eat animal protein a few times per week, rather than every day. Our planet would benefit if you limited your animal protein intake. If you are a vegetarian, you'll eat legumes for both servings every day. There are key macro- and micro-nutrients in protein, such as amino acids, that we need for balancing our chemical messengers. It's important to choose clean sources—that is, proteins that are organic, free range, pasture raised, and grass fed.

* Grains: One or more servings per day. A general serving size is 1 cup cooked grains, one slice of bread, or one tortilla. Some days or seasons you may choose to go grain-free, and that's perfectly healthy if you are getting your minimum servings of vegetables and fruit. During certain times of the year when grains are more abundant and other food sources are scarce, grains can be a good source of nourishment. I will delve into which grains are best to consume and when.

* Oils: The quantity depends on how much you get in plant and animal sources, but typically you'll want to add in at least three servings with your dressings and sauces, as well as when baking and cooking. A general serving size is 1 tablespoon. The key here is the type of oil and when to use it. Certain oils, like avocado oil, can handle higher temperatures, whereas others, like olive oil, are best used outside of cooking, such as in dressings.

* Herbs and spices: Two or more servings per day. A general serving size is about 1 teaspoon of spices and 1 tablespoon of herbs, but it depends on the herb or spice and how much flavor you want to add. Herbs and spices add flavor to our food and have health benefits as well. For example, cinnamon is known to help balance blood sugar, and turmeric is known for its anti-inflammatory effects.

* Liquids: 2.5 to 3.0 liters daily (non-caffeinated). The ones I encourage you to focus on include filtered water (year-round), herbal teas (warm in fall and winter and chilled or room temp in spring and summer) as well as smoothies (chilled in spring and summer and cool to room temperature in fall and winter) and fresh seasonal juices.

* Sweeteners: While you can skip these, I knew you'd ask! And I don't blame you. I like the occasional treat as well. I will share which are the best sweeteners to enjoy at various times of the year.

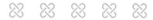

Preprogram Tips to Help Set You Up for Success

* Write down your health, skin, and other lifestyle goals.
* Plan your menus, make your shopping lists, and schedule your meals before you start each phase of the program.
* Note in your journal how you feel after eating each season's meals. Some foods

may feel more energizing or satisfying than others, so you'll be able to reflect back and see which foods gave your energy a boost or were more comforting.

❖ If you have an eating disorder or emotional triggers around eating, discuss this program with your healthcare provider before starting it.

MOVEMENT BASICS FOR ALL SEASONS

Exercise isn't one-size-fits-all. Depending on your unique DNA, not to mention your goals, exercise type, intensity, and frequency will vary. Beyond that, exercise needs tend to change throughout life as well as throughout the seasons.

Exercise leads to perspiration, which is one of the easiest ways to get toxins out of the body. A study published in *Scientific World Journal* showed the presence of phthalate metabolites in the samples of the twenty participants' sweat, showing that perspiring can be an effective way to eliminate toxic phthalate compounds from the body.[97] In the warmer months, it's easier to perspire, but if your fall and winter is cold, it may be harder to break a sweat. It is important to sweat regularly—at least once per week, so plan your routine accordingly.

Yoga is a form of movement that also includes mindset. Meditation with yoga may help reduce the rate of cellular aging, suggests a twelve-week study.[98] You don't have to be a yogi to enjoy the benefits of

yoga, and I'll share yoga poses to try out for each season. You can follow along in an online (such as on YouTube) or in-person yoga class to get the most out of these therapeutic poses.

If you're new to exercise or it's been a while since you've worked out regularly, ease your way in. Also, if you're recovering from an injury or have a medical condition, check with your doctor before starting a new fitness activity or dramatically altering your routine.

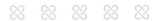

Preprogram Tips to Help Set You Up for Success

❖ Write down your goals for fitness.
❖ Plan ahead and create your movement routine for the initial seven days of each season.
❖ Note in your journal how you feel after each season's movement routine so you'll be able to reflect on how you may be able to use movement to give you a boost or help you unwind.
❖ If you have physical limitations, injuries, or health conditions that impact your ability to move, remember to talk to your doctor.

MINDSET BASICS FOR ALL SEASONS

Beauty is more than a physical description; it's a state of mind. Our mindset and the choices we make each day are what helps our authentic beauty evolve and shine. We can choose to be kind, compassionate, authentic, bold, and loving without losing our power or our identity.

It's not always easy, though, because life throws challenges our way—from work and our social lives to health and homelife situations. Our thoughts can be toxic and block our path to confidence and natural beauty. Added to that, negative thoughts and unmanaged stress puts a burden on our adrenals and nervous systems, which creates a number of hormonal imbalances that perpetuate harmful misbeliefs and behaviors. The good news is that mindfulness practices are free and available to you 24/7!

In each season's mindset section, you'll learn ways to adopt a daily practice for stress management and mindfulness to help reset your beliefs, reprogram your self-talk, and rebalance your chemical messengers. Practices include specific examples of mindfulness exercises such as meditation and breathwork, as well as nature excursions. Breathwork helps cleanse the mind as well as the body. Our lungs are one of our underrecognized pathways of detoxification, so we want to include regular breathwork for both body and mind.

A boon to the mind is sleep, which is also essential for vibrant-looking skin as we age. For example, melatonin, the hormone our bodies release that signals it's time for sleep, contains metabolites that have protective actions for the skin. These metabolites protect against diseases,

including cancer and inflammatory conditions as well as against the insults of UV radiation exposure. You can refer to year-round sleep tips in chapter 4 to help support your melatonin production and restorative sleep.

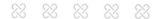

Preprogram Tips to Help Set You Up for Success

* Write down your goals for your mood and mindset.
* Plan ahead and create your mindset routine for the initial seven days of each season.
* When you come across ideas you want to rid yourself of (negative thoughts), use loose-leaf paper and shred or burn these safely, such as in a fireplace or firepit. In your journal, keep only positive thoughts, affirmations, and feelings of gratitude that raise your awareness of the positives in your life. This will help you release that which no longer serves you (by burning or shredding) and keep the words that are helping you restore beauty and balance.

SKINCARE BASICS FOR ALL SEASONS

As we turn our attention to our body's largest organ, let's remember to be kind to our skin, which is our biggest defender against the outside world. We are often too quick to tap into many modern-day conveniences that promise quick fixes (skincare products with toxic ingredients) or conceal perceived blemishes (makeup).

The goals of this program include supporting the skin's ideal pH, nourishing the barrier function of the microbiota, de-stressing the skin, aiding hormonal balance throughout the body, and making smart choices when it comes to choosing skincare products and ingredients. As a result, you will be able to decrease inflammation in the body and slow collagen loss, thereby keeping blemishes, eruptions, and signs of premature aging at bay.

Beware of potential toxins. As women, we tend to use more beauty products as we get older, which is tricky because this is often when our hormones begin to fluctuate more. Remember that many skincare products contain EDCs, which have been linked to fertility issues, irregular menses, breast cancer, thyroid disease, and neuroendocrine problems, to name a few. Some ingredients are not listed on the label or are listed by their complex chemical names, which prevents us from knowing what we're really exposing our skin to, so refer to the skincare ingredient list in chapter 10.

Understand pH and your skin. Using topical products with an ideal pH helps support the skin's natural barrier function, including a healthy skin microbiome. As we discussed in chapter 2, you can support your skin's pH and nourish your skin microbiome by using skincare products with a pH of 4.6 to 5.4 and key natural actives.

Take steps to de-stress your skin. Choosing topical agents that have balancing effects can help de-stress the skin. Research has demonstrated that skin is impacted not only by psychological stress, but also by a stress response in the local HPA axis in the skin, peripheral nerve endings, and local skin cells, including keratinocytes, mast cells, and immune cells. Stress has a direct effect on the skin, causing the production of stress hormones and inflammatory factors.[99]

While we need further research to understand how topical substances may be able to impact the HPA axis in the skin, at least one study suggests that they have the potential to affect the skin's stress response.[100] There are natural substances called adaptogenic herbs, such as rhodiola, ashwagandha, astragalus, and ginseng, that are known to have a balancing effect on the stress response and that may work topically as well.

Don't skimp on quality sunscreen. While sunscreen is key for reducing the risk of skin cancer and warding off wrinkles, some products are preferable to others. It's important to understand how the SPF and ingredients in your sunscreen are working. First, know that no sunscreen can 100 percent protect you from the sun's rays.

An SPF of 15 gives you a 93 percent blockage from Ultraviolet B (UVB) rays, an SPF of 30 gives you a 97 percent, and an SPF of 50 gives you a 98 percent blockage from UVB rays. (Anything with an SPF of above 50 doesn't offer additional protective benefits and is just marketing hype.)

But SPF is only a measurement of protection from the UVB rays, which are the burning rays. We also are exposed to the Ultraviolet A (UVA) rays, which are the aging rays that come through window glass and don't vary throughout the year. If you're wearing sunscreen and you're not getting burned, that doesn't mean you're not getting damaged by the sun. In fact, research shows UVA can be a significant factor in tumor initiation as well as tumor promotion.[101]

You need 2 tablespoons of sunblock for your whole body, and a nickel-size amount for your face is a good rule of thumb. Don't forget to reapply every two hours.

Some of the chemicals in sunscreen, such as oxybenzone, have been linked to hormone-disrupting effects. I recommend buying a mineral-based sunscreen made with zinc oxide and using protective clothing, hats, and sunglasses.

Don't overthink your skincare routine. It can be similar both morning and night, and you do need both to revitalize skin in the morning and to clean and nourish it before bedtime. While there are many natural skincare lines on the market today, most do not meet my criteria. I created The Spa Dr. skincare line to embrace these practices and principles and to provide an easy system for you.

For each season, I will provide recommendations on ingredients and skincare routines, but first, keep the basics in mind.

Namely, a nourishing skincare routine is one that:

- is free of toxins,
- contains natural actives that allow for healing and graceful aging, and
- is pH-perfected to be mildly acidic.

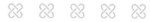

Preprogram Tips to Help Set You Up for Success

- Take a "before" picture of your skin and write down your skincare goals.
- Plan ahead with DIY skincare recipes and recommendations for the initial seven days of each season.
- At the end of every seasonal seven-day reset, look at your magic mirror (your skin) and take note of what you see. Snap an "after" picture and compare it to the "before" picture you took before you started the program. Make sure the picture is as close to the same lighting and setting as your first picture so you can get a true comparison.
- Note in your journal how your skin looks and feels after each season's skincare practices so you'll be able to reflect on which worked best for your skin.
- If you have chronic skin issues or an acute skin problem arises, check with your dermatologist, naturopathic doctor, and/or aesthetician for individualized support.

CHAPTER 8

FALL
RESET

(September, October, and November)

Life starts all over again
when it gets crisp in the fall.

—F. Scott Fitzgerald

Fall is a time of transition from the warm, sunny days of summer. The fall equinox is the date when day and night are equal in length, so starting the fall seven-day reset around this time is ideal. In the northern hemisphere, this happens from the 21st to the 24th of September, while in the southern hemisphere it occurs in March. The day after the fall equinox is when nights become longer until we get to the spring equinox, when the nights become shorter.

In fall, as we shift away from a bustling summer and prepare our bodies for winter, we may feel the changes that occur with the sun. Many women experience more PMS in cooler months, and seasonal affective disorder (SAD) starts to set in for many. Preparing for this time of year means supporting your mood as well as a healthy immune system before cold and flu season begins.

The Natural Beauty Reset will put you one step ahead of these changes so your body can restore its natural rhythms and harmonize its hormones. The first season you do this program may be the most challenging, especially if you are currently experiencing symptoms such as difficulty falling or staying asleep, irregular menstrual cycles, night sweats, challenges with losing or gaining weight, or morning fatigue.

There is a correlation between less sunlight and hormonal shifts. For instance, the darker days of autumn cause a drop in serotonin, so you may not feel as positive as you did in the summer. If you're prone to excess sadness (which is, of course, a normal emotion), you can get ahead of the winter blues with the fall reset. If you do experience SAD or another mental health disorder, now is a great time to check in with your doctor to evaluate your hormones, as well as with a mental health specialist, both of whom can provide you with additional support and guidance for the season.

A shift can happen with thyroid hormones in the fall. If you notice low mood, fatigue, weight gain, intolerance to cold, and brain fog, check in with your doctor and get your thyroid panel (TSH, free T3, free T4, and thyroid antibodies). Wintertime can cause natural shifts to these hormones. For instance, the active thyroid hormone T3 may be higher in response to cold this time of year compared to the summer.[102] It's good to get your blood work done before the weather turns cooler, so you have a baseline to go from.

Due to heightened levels of stress this time of year, keep in mind that you may be more prone to reach for comfort foods.

Instead of suppressing these desires, succumb to savory or sweet food urges with deliciously nutritious foods instead of highly processed comfort foods. As energy and metabolism may slow a bit in fall compared to summer and you're likely spending more time indoors, it's helpful to be mindful of your food and movement choices.

Less sun exposure in fall also means vitamin D stores may wane. Vitamin D deficiency impacts 50 percent of the global population—nearly 1 billion people of different ages and ethnicities.[103] To avoid being a part of this statistic, get your 25-hydroxy vitamin D levels tested. You recently enjoyed a boost in your sun exposure and are on the brink of the darker days of winter, so you want to check your levels to make sure they're high enough to last through the less sunny months ahead. If they're low or on the lower end of the normal range, it's a good time to start taking a vitamin D_3 supplement. The dosage of vitamin D_3 depends on your needs, but, in general, 2,000 IU daily is a great place to start, or closer to 10,000 IU daily or 50,000 IU weekly if your levels are low.[104]

Hormonally speaking, one bright spot of fall is that darker days typically lead to higher testosterone levels. In fact, some experts believe that testosterone is highest in the autumn because of higher vitamin D levels in the summer, which triggers testosterone production. With higher testosterone levels, you may find you have higher libido and overall motivation, and you may find it easier to gain muscle with your exercise routine.

Another perk as we shift toward more darkness is that our melatonin levels start to increase (compared to spring and summer), so sleep may be easier.[105] If you currently struggle with sleep, this season is a good time to get your sleep back on track as you have darkness on your side (in a good way!). The downside of this is we may start to feel drowsier during the day compared to summer, as the days are shorter and melatonin production will naturally increase as the darkness sets in earlier.

Now, let's dive into the specifics of the 7-Day Fall Reset to help you adjust to these changes.

Fall Food

Fall harvest brings produce that is long-lasting and heartier than summer's. Because there is less opportunity for spoilage, your shopping may also be less expensive. If you have a garden, transition it because this is the time of harvest.

We want to consume nutritionally dense foods to protect our immune systems going into winter. Eating foods in season is a wise way to do that. Choose foods high in nutrients such as zinc, vitamin C, vitamin A, and B vitamins (including B_{12}, B_6, folate, and thiamine) because these are associated with immune health. Leafy greens (like collard greens, kale, and frisée), bell peppers, and cruciferous vegetables (such as broccoli, cauliflower, cabbage, brussels sprouts, turnips, and bok choy) are some of the top veggies to eat this time of year to help give your mood and immune system a boost.

These nutrients, along with omega-3 fatty acids (EPA and DHA), iron, magnesium, potassium, and selenium, may also help protect against depression.[106] Foods in season containing these nutrients include pacific halibut, free-range turkey, kale, lentils, green beans, almonds, chia seeds, sunflower kernels, and pecans.

Remember that 90 percent of serotonin receptors are actually in the gut, so what you eat does make a difference in mood. Eating an anti-inflammatory diet has been shown to help protect against depression, and eating high-fiber foods helps support a healthy gut microbiome.[107] All of this can be achieved with the recommended fall food list and recipes in this section.

Serotonin is made from tryptophan, which is mostly found in high-protein foods such as fish, poultry, and meat. But we need carbohydrates to help with the mood-stabilizing effects. Eating carbs increases insulin, which helps with amino acid absorption.

While you may crave sugar, eating the sweet stuff is known to actually decrease serotonin.[108] So you'll want to find healthier comfort foods to help adjust for possible drops in serotonin during the cooler months. Since fruit is a more nourishing substitute to processed sugar, you can enjoy fall produce such as pears, apples, and figs and avoid cooling, out-of-season fruit like watermelon.

If you're not a sweets person but are instead partial to crunchy, salty, or cheesy food for comfort, seek out nutrient-dense options such as my kale chip recipe, a nut mix, or a delicious bean dip. Doing so will help keep your gut health in good shape and your blood sugar steady.

Ideally, look at both short- and long-term solutions for your meal plan. For example, cinnamon is a great spice to include in cooler months because it adds a sweet flavor while having a blood sugar–balancing effect and warming properties.

For additional seasonal foods, check with your local farmers market to find out which produce is freshest where you live. Choose organic, local, and nongenetically modified food as much as possible.

Foods most abundant during fall include:

❉ Grains: These grains are typically harvested in late summer into fall. Grains can be found year-round, but I include them here because they're freshest. Grains, like all food, are perishable so it's best to store them in a cool, dry place, or, in the case of flours, in the refrigerator to ensure freshness.

AMARANTH	CORN (NON-GMO)	OATS
BASMATI RICE	MILLET	QUINOA

❉ Fruits: Since fruit is less plentiful in fall, our focus shifts more to vegetables, which are abundant this time of year.

APPLES	GOJI BERRIES	PEARS
CRAB APPLES	GRAPES	PERSIMMONS
CRANBERRIES	KEY LIMES	POMEGRANATES
FIGS	KIWIS	QUINCES

❖ Vegetables: Fall harvest brings in a vast array of vegetables. Check with your local farmers for the freshest varieties available in your current month.

ARUGULA	CHARD	PUMPKINS
BEETS	COLLARD GREENS	RADICCHIOS
BELL PEPPERS	EGGPLANTS	RADISHES
BOK CHOY	ESCAROLE	RUTABAGAS
BROCCOLI RABE	FRISÉE	SPINACH
BRUSSELS SPROUTS	KALE	SUNCHOKES
BURDOCKS	LEEKS	SWEET POTATOES
CABBAGES	OLIVES	AND YAMS
CARROTS	PARSNIPS	TURNIPS
CAULIFLOWER	POTATOES	WILD MUSHROOMS
CELERY	(yellow, blue, and red)	(besides morel)
		WINTER SQUASH

❖ Legumes: While they can be found year-round, these legumes are more abundant in fall compared to other legumes.

EDAMAME	GREEN BEANS	LENTILS

❖ Nuts and seeds: Nuts can be enjoyed year-round, but their oils can become rancid so it's best to enjoy them as fresh as possible and to store them in dry, cool locations.

ALMONDS	HAZELNUTS	PISTACHIOS
BUTTERNUTS	PECANS	SUNFLOWER
CHIA SEEDS	PINE NUTS	KERNELS
		WALNUTS

❋ Animal protein: Animals have seasons, too. You'll find these animal proteins are easiest to find in fall.

TURKEY   WILD, LINE-CAUGHT
                      PACIFIC HALIBUT

❋ Herbs and spices: These herbs and spices create the flavors of fall because this is the time when they're typically easiest to grow.

CHICORIES   GINGER   ROSEMARY
CHILES   ONIONS   SAGE
FENNEL   (red, yellow, and white)   THYME
GARLIC   PARSLEY

❋ Sweets: You can skip the sweets if you prefer, but if you want an occasional indulgence, these are your seasonal best and are more nutritious than processed sugar.

DATES   HONEY

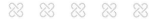

Many other foods from around the world are abundant in fall months and available to us, but these are examples of foods to focus on as you're planning your seven-day reset.

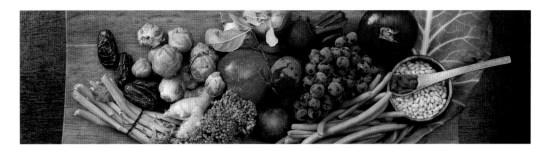

SAMPLE FALL MEAL
IDEAS FROM RECIPES

Here are a week's worth of ideas to help you get started on the 7-Day Natural Beauty Reset for fall. Feel free to modify, substitute, and repeat recipes throughout. Remember, this is not about restriction or limitations; it's about enjoying the flavors and nourishment available during the season you're in. Make note of which meals you like best so you can continue making them throughout the fall season.

SAMPLE DAY 1

BREAKFAST: Pumpkin Spice Smoothie (page 151)

LUNCH: White Bean Soup with Collard Greens (page 157)

DINNER: Halibut Tacos with Red Cabbage Slaw (page 153)

SNACKS/SWEETS: Cinnamon Oat Bites (page 168)

SAMPLE DAY 2

BREAKFAST: Ultimate Green Smoothie Juice (page 153)

LUNCH: Turkey Meatballs with Parsley Pesto and Zucchini Pasta (page 155)

DINNER: Quinoa Lentil Salad with Roasted Eggplant (page 158)

SNACKS/SWEETS: Kale Chips (page 171)

SAMPLE DAY 3

BREAKFAST: Overnight Chia Oats (page 152)

LUNCH: Roasted Brussels Sprouts and Apple Salad (page 164)

DINNER: Lime Chili Halibut with Garlic Kale (page 160)

SNACKS/SWEETS: Pumpkin Pie with Almond Crust (page 170)

SAMPLE DAY 4

BREAKFAST: Ginger Chia Pudding with Pomegranate Seeds (page 152)

LUNCH: Creamy Broccoli Soup (page 161)

DINNER: Black Bean Turkey Chili (page 162)

SNACKS/SWEETS: Chocolate Truffles (page 169)

SAMPLE DAY 5

BREAKFAST: Make your own smoothie bowl with one serving of seasonal fruit, one serving of fall greens, 1 cup of almond or hazelnut milk, and one serving of seasonal nuts or protein powder (optional: add fresh ginger for seasonal flavor)

LUNCH: Leftover Black Bean Turkey Chili

DINNER: Make your own quinoa salad with edamame beans and any of the following: cabbage, bell peppers, bok choy, fennel, chard, carrots, kale, escarole, leeks, spinach, collard greens, radishes, brussels sprouts, winter squash, and olives

SNACKS/SWEETS: Make your own snack by mixing one sliced organic apple with 2 tablespoons almond butter

TIP: Find ways to maximize your time and minimize prep. For example, make more than the recipe calls for and set aside as leftovers or chop a few days' worth of vegetables and fruit and store in a glass or ceramic container in the refrigerator

SAMPLE DAY 6

BREAKFAST: Cinnamon Granola (see winter recipe on page 173) with unsweetened almond or hazelnut milk

LUNCH: Fall Harvest Salad (page 166) topped with sliced turkey breast

DINNER: Red Lentil Soup (page 163)

SNACKS/SWEETS: Beau Pa's Cookies (page 167)

SAMPLE DAY 7

BREAKFAST: Make your own breakfast with two turkey sausage patties (nitrate free) and roasted seasonal veggies

LUNCH: Leftover Red Lentil Soup

DINNER: Make your own dinner with roasted cauliflower, brussels sprouts (or other seasonal veggies), and baked or grilled halibut

SNACKS/SWEETS: Fig Pudding (use the Ginger Chia Pudding with Pomegranate Seeds recipe [page 152] but use fresh figs instead of fruit)

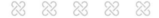

ADDITIONAL SNACK IDEAS FOR FALL

- Rooibos chai tea latte with almond milk
- Edamame (steamed with sea salt)
- Mixed nuts (any combination of pistachios, almonds, sunflower seeds, pecans, pine nuts, hazelnuts, or walnuts)
- Roasted pumpkin seeds
- Apple sauce with a dash of cinnamon
- Fruit salad (any combination of apples, figs, pomegranates, pears, grapes, persimmons, quinces, or kiwis)

Fall Movement

With the shift into fall, your body may crave more rest and less activity. But that doesn't mean you can't enjoy all that the season has to offer, such as the changing colors of the leaves. Try hiking, taking walks in the park, or biking for gentle exercise.

If you experience changes in your mood with your cycle or have been diagnosed with premenstrual dysphoric disorder (PMDD)—a very severe form of premenstrual syndrome (PMS)—or seasonal affective disorder (SAD), pay close attention to the exercises in this section to help keep your energy and mood high. It's best to start these before you have symptoms, but it's never too late to begin making changes.

A significant focus during fall is preparing for winter, which is a time when mood tends to decline. Fortunately, exercise offers an easy solution. But don't overdo it—moderation is key, research shows.

In a study published in *Lancet* that looked at patterns of mental health burden and exercise of 1.2 million people, researchers found those who exercised reported an average of 43 percent fewer days of poor mental health than those who didn't exercise.[109] Any type and frequency of exercise was a boon to the participants' mood. Participants who moved for forty-five minutes three to five times a week and played popular team sports, cycled, and did aerobic and gym exercise saw the biggest mood lift.

Since women typically have higher testosterone levels in summer and fall, this is an ideal time of year to renew or get a gym membership and begin pumping some iron.[110] That elevated testosterone in the fall means building muscle will be easier than in other times of year. If going to a gym sounds too daunting, try creating a home gym. A jump rope and trampoline are examples of affordable cardio equipment to keep handy, while resistance bands, physio balls, and lightweight dumbbells (think 3 to 10 pounds) can help you build strength. If you want to go equipment-free, there are plenty of body-weight-bearing exercises you can try. Turn to the web for app and workout equipment ideas as well as plenty of inspiration to stick to your home workout.

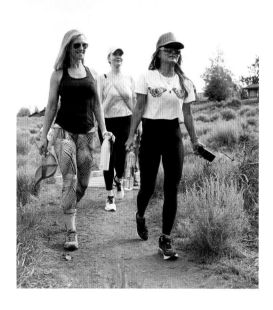

While a home workout can be efficient, easy, and cost-effective, I also encourage you to connect with a community for keeping active. You can attend fitness classes and show up early to connect with others. Or invite people to join you on a fall hike or bike ride. Here's why: When we are feeling stressed, sad, or anxious, it's harder to connect with others socially, which can worsen these unpleasant feelings. The potential result is a vicious cycle of pulling back from the very things that help us feel happier and more connected. Fall is the perfect time to find and solidify your community. This way, when the heaviness of the winter blues sets in, you have a group of people to help lift your spirits.

Here are examples of movements for each of the seven days of your fall reset. You can choose to do one each day or pick three or four to complete throughout the week. After a week of trying these exercises, you can continue your favorites throughout the fall season. And before we dive in, note that if you have physical limitations or injuries or a medical condition, consult with your healthcare provider before dramatically changing your workout routine.

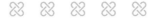

7 Movements for Fall

1. **Take a fall hike or bike ride.**
   Fall is an ideal time for hiking and biking because the temperatures tend to be cooler, and if you live in a place where the leaves change colors, it's a great opportunity to take in the beauty of the season. This type of movement improves balance and helps strengthen and tone muscles throughout the body. Being in the great outdoors also helps manage stress and boosts mood.

   Take advantage of the weather and prepare with the right clothing. Bring a small backpack with water, a windbreaker, and sunscreen. If you can, grab a friend or go with a group, and work on strengthening your bonds with others.

2. **Enjoy a fitness class or outdoor sport.**
   Have fun with this. Try taking a fitness or dance class, or gather some family and friends and a soccer ball and head to your local park. This activity is meant to be fun and creative to help lift your spirits along with your heart rate.

   If you're bored with your fitness class, try taking a different one. Sometimes doing something new can feel like a daunting task, but I encourage you to muster the courage to take the leap and keep an open mind. I've been to so many fitness classes—some I've loved, and some I just managed to get through. Classes that encourage creativity like dancing can feel so fun that it doesn't feel like exercise, and a great instructor can help you forget the time and fall back in love with the way your body moves.

If sports are more your jam yet you still want that structure and company a class provides, consider signing up for a club sport or taking lessons for activities like pickleball, tennis, volleyball, or soccer.

3. **Set up a buddy workout.**
Having a friend join you for a workout makes the time pass more quickly. I've had some of the deepest philosophical conversations with my personal trainer and friend during a fitness routine in my home or neighborhood gym. If you're new to working out, I encourage you to find a friend who can help keep you motivated. For tips on form and performance, consider hiring a personal trainer who can create a routine that you can follow on your own.

4. **Try tai chi, qigong, or dance.**
If you haven't heard of tai chi or qigong, you're missing out! These ancient Chinese traditions are known for helping people relieve stress and restore or revitalize energy. Tai chi is sometimes referred to as meditation in motion and is a form of martial arts that involves a series of slow-moving, mindful moves. Qigong, meanwhile, is a system of wellness that combines movement, breathing, and meditative practice to help with a mind-body-spirit connection.

People of all ages and fitness levels can enjoy these activities. You do not have to subscribe to a particular spiritual or philosophical belief system to participate in these activities. To enjoy these Chinese practices, find an online or in-person program or class, and take your time exploring the healing benefits.

If you're not ready or able to do these, turn up some music at home and dance. Move your body slowly and rhythmically while being conscious of your breathing, and let your thoughts go out the window as you focus on your body and how healing is available to you.

5. **Create your own home circuit.**
Home circuits are perfect for the busy woman looking for a short yet effective workout. I suggest doing this in the morning so you can check it off your list and feel revitalized for the remainder of the day. However, if evening is your only time, that's okay. Just be sure to complete the routine at least a few hours before bedtime so that your body and mind have time to shift into relaxation mode.

This is a six-minute routine that can be repeated as your time allows. Each exercise takes one minute to complete. I recommend doing this routine three to five times a week.

❋ Jog or march in place or jump rope (if you have knee or other joint issues or want a lower-impact version, choose marching in place)

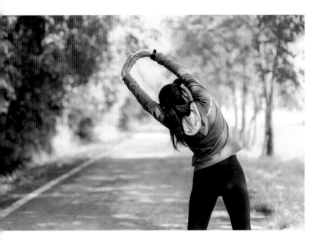

- Alternating lunges (lunge forward alternating legs if space allows, or lunge in place by stepping back into a lunge with alternating legs)
- High-knee jog or march (if you have knee or other joint issues, or want a lower-impact version, choose marching in place while lifting your knees high in front of you)
- Squat kicks (just as it sounds, squat and then kick out with alternating legs)
- Jumping jacks (remember PE class from school? Yep, just like that! For a lower-impact version, instead of jumping, step back in place, alternating each foot)
- Squat jumps (squat and then jump. For a lower-impact version, stand instead of jump and then squat again)

6. **Select some grounding yoga poses.** Choose poses that are grounding to help you reconnect with the earth. Yoga has gained popularity around the world, and for good reason! Its practices are easily modifiable and aim to improve flexibility, making these mindful exercises great options for people of all ages and fitness levels. You can do simple poses almost anywhere, anytime. Here are a few of my favorites for fall to help restore balance and stretch commonly tense areas of the body. To learn how to do these therapeutic poses and to get the most out of them, I recommend taking a video or an in-person yoga class.

- Forward fold: This pose calms the mind while stretching the hamstrings (the major muscles at the upper back part of your legs) and back.
- Extended side angle: This pose focuses on balance, breathing, and stretching the side of the body.
- Warrior I and II: These poses help with balance and strengthening your legs, while stretching muscles around your hips.
- Savasana: A relaxation pose that calms the mind and brings about deep awareness.

7. **Do yard work or take a walk in the park.** If you live in a place where the leaves drop, now is the perfect time to rake them, which will leave you with a clear lawn and a great workout. If you don't have a yard, see if there is a neighborhood elder who would love the extra help.

A walk in your nearby park is a great option for enjoying the health benefits of nature. Much research has shown the mental health effects of spending time in nature. One study showed that people who walked in nature for ninety minutes (compared to those who walk in high-traffic urban areas) had experienced less rumination (repetitive negative thoughts) and decreased activity in the area of the brain associated with risk for depression.[111] If that study alone is not enough to get you in nature for a walk, dogs are a great motivator. If you don't have a dog, ask a friend or neighbor if you can walk their dog once per week, or volunteer at your local pet shelter. Having a companion for a walk, whether it's a dog or human, is a great way to enjoy this movement even further.

Fall Mindset

This time of year, the plants prepare for winter. Leaves fall and frost covers the ground as temperatures drop. As the leaves fall, we, too, have the opportunity to drop negative thoughts and beliefs that we no longer need. This season helps us prepare for what is ahead in the coming months and the neurochemical shifts we may experience with the change of seasons.

To keep our mood and mojo elevated, we want to shift our mindset practices. Our focus can turn inward more. Coming off the creativity and abundance of summer, fall is an ideal season to reevaluate our projects, recall what's truly important, and clean up our to-do lists.

Fall is also a good time to start bringing the outside in. We can set ourselves up for winter with creativity and preparing our homes to be happy, healthy havens. As we watch leaves change and the outdoors transform, it is an opportune time to notice the transformation happening within us.

Studies have indicated that time in nature (when people feel safe) helps alleviate stress, increase self-esteem, reduce anxiety, and improve mood.[112] So I encourage you to stay connected with nature even when cooler temperatures are upon us and plants are less abundant. We may not feel as motivated to step outdoors, but our bodies still crave this connection. Creating a routine and having the right gear can help set you up for success.

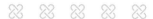

7 Mindset Activities for Fall

1. **Release and reflect through journaling.**

❃ Review and record thoughts and emotions that may be holding you back so that you can start to release them from your life. As seasons change, it's an opportunity to press the reset button and reprogram our belief systems. A study published by Cambridge University showed that writing to express your emotions for fifteen to twenty minutes can help improve immune function, mood, memory, and performance.[113] If your thoughts feel heavy, they're likely holding you back and can interfere with your healing journey. Why carry around that extra weight when you can move forward more easily without it?

On a piece of loose paper, make a list of everything in your life that feels like a burden, a weight, or an obstacle in your healing journey. Take your time as you write each item down and notice how your body feels. Do you feel heaviness, pain, or discomfort? Where do you feel it? Once you've written your list, burn or shred the paper and feel those burdens being lifted away.

❁ Take time for reflection. In your journal, take stock of your life in the current moment. Do this simply and without judgment as if you're a neutral observer of your life. It's easy to be a critic, but can you simply reflect? What did you notice in your body and mind when burning the list of burdens? Did you notice a shift? How can you move forward on a more positive foot without those distractions?

2. **Try out breathwork for transition.** Alternating nostril breathwork in particular helps us restore balance, quiet the mind, and create a sense of calm. A simple alternative nostril-breathing exercise

is to exhale all the air out of your lungs. With your right-hand ring finger, close the left nostril and inhale through the right nostril. Then close the right nostril with your right-hand thumb. Exhale through the left nostril and then inhale through the left, then close the left nostril with your ring finger and exhale through the right. Repeat ten times.

3. **Do a mantra meditation or prayer.** Prayer and meditation are opportunities to quiet negative internal dialogue and improve our sense of well-being. If you already have a meditation or prayer practice that works well for you, that's great! If you don't, I encourage you to try a few options. Regardless of your religious or spiritual belief system, you can gain great benefit from taking a few minutes to a few hours for a prayer or meditation practice. Research shows spiritual practice can decrease anxiety and depression and help boost melatonin and serotonin and lower cortisol.[114]

A prayer can be as simple as asking for guidance and expressing gratitude. And a mantra meditation can start with silently repeating a positive sound, word, or statement. This can be something simple like *peace* or *I am enough* or a sacred word that ties into your religious or spiritual belief system. For example, *Sat Nam* and *Om Shanti Om* are commonly used mantras in yoga practice. Start by setting an intention before your practice, sit upright in a quiet, comfortable place, close your eyes, and repeat your mantra for as long as you'd like or until you feel a sense of quiet in your mind.

4. **Connect with your community.**
Finding and connecting with like-minded individuals can help ease stress and give you a sense of belonging. Feeling isolated and alone can suppress your immune system, so it's important to spend time with your community in the fall. Getting outdoors with friends and family can offer the benefits of connecting with nature.

5. **Get creative for fall.**
Participating in creative activities can have benefits similar to meditating, giving your mind a break from ruminating thoughts and helping you achieve a sense of well-being. This time of year, you can get crafty with art projects or tap into your creativity in the kitchen. For example, take some of your summer produce and can or dry it to use in the cooler months ahead. Those cucumbers from your local farmers market are a yummy source for bright pickles, and that fall cabbage is a few steps away from becoming sauerkraut, which will add an extra bite to your meals ahead. Go to your local apple orchard to pick apples and dry them so you can have a tasty, healthy snack on the go.

6. **Look for ways to bring more light and nature into your home.**
Light exposure during the day helps our circadian rhythm, which in turn impacts our mood and sleep. Since fall is darker than summer, we want to find ways to improve light exposure this time of year. The best time of day for light exposure is early morning. Natural daytime light, as opposed to nighttime light, exposure makes a difference in our mood and sleep.

According to a study in *Sleep Health* of 109 participants, office workers exposed to light in the morning had less difficulty falling asleep and better sleep quality than those who didn't have much light exposure during the morning hours.[115] Those exposed to light during daytime hours experienced a reduction in depression.

To help your light exposure, you can go outdoors in the morning or stand near a sunny window. Natural light is the best, but if the weather is overcast, you can also use artificial light. If the area where you live is often cloudy or overcast during the fall and winter months, you may want to consider getting a light therapy lamp, which mimics outdoor light by emitting a broad-spectrum ultraviolet light. The most common prescription is thirty minutes of usage at the beginning of every morning, with the box or lamp 12 to 24 inches away.

7. **Limit your screen time and consider blue light blockers.**

As you shift from summer to fall, you may be spending more time on your electronic devices. With this comes greater exposure to blue light. While some blue light is natural (from the sun) and can boost our alertness, today, most of us get too much exposure to blue light–emitting devices like cell phones, computers, electronic readers, and TVs. You may also want to consider blue-light-blocking glasses to moderate melatonin production for optimal sleep.

Fall Skincare

Fluctuating daytime temperatures combined with cool winds are a recipe for dry, irritated skin. Coming off summertime, your skin is recovering from the harsh sun, and after a season of perspiring, you may notice your pores are larger than usual.

You may consider turning to restorative facials to help soothe sun damage and rehydrate your skin. This can also be a fun time to take some of the seasonal foods from your plate and incorporate them into your skincare routine for nourishing, natural remedies. For example, you might try the DIY Pumpkin Face Mask or the Chia, Honey, and Green Tea Face Wash. (Find instructions for both in the recipes section, page 225.)

Here are seven skincare practices to incorporate in your Fall Natural Beauty Reset. You can choose one per day or choose several to repeat throughout the week. Note your favorites and continue using them through the fall season.

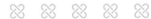

7 Skincare Practices for Fall

1. **Bump up the hydration in your moisturizers.**

Look for moisturizers for your face and body that include naturally derived hydrating ingredients such as hyaluronate, niacinamide, glycerin, and plant-based oils such as pomegranate seed oil, cranberry seed oil, and apricot kernel oil.[116] Avoid mineral oil and other petroleum-based synthetic ingredients that may feel lightly hydrating but lack the same kind of nutritional enrichment as plant-based oils. You want to look and feel hydrated but not gooey and sticky.

For DIY cleansers, steams, and masks, include ingredients such as honey, coconut oil, oats, and essential oils such as lavender and ylang-ylang. (Note: because essential oils are highly concentrated, be sure to use caution around pets and young children.) For extra skin-pampering hydration, apply body lotion after stepping out of the shower or bath while your skin is still damp and then gently pat your skin with a towel.

2. **Use a hydrating cleanser and skip the toner.**

Start your skincare routine using a cleanser with plant-based oils such as jojoba, argan, or almond. Avoid high-pH cleansers, like those that make suds and foam. If you're not sure of the pH, simply use a pH strip and check for yourself. If you choose a cleanser that fits this description, you won't need a toner. Because they often contain alcohol and astringents, toners can be drying to the skin, which you do not need in fall months. Toners are typically designed to tighten the skin and remove residual dirt, pollutants, and impurities on the skin that remain after cleansing. If you're feeling the need for a toner after cleansing your face because your face still feels oily, try changing your cleanser first, then follow that with a highly nourishing antioxidant-rich serum.

3. **Bump up the antioxidants.**

To help soothe damage from a summer of sun and outdoor air pollutants contacting your skin, look for skincare with high-antioxidant ingredients such as resveratrol, green algae extract, turmeric, and green, black, white, and rooibos teas. To create DIY options, look to seasonal foods high in antioxidants such as pumpkin, apples, pomegranates, grapes, chia seeds, honey, chard, and kale. The recipes section is bursting with ideas featuring these fall staples.

4. **Exfoliate gently and with care.**

With the change of seasons to cooler months, and especially if you tend toward dryer skin, reduce or eliminate the use of more intense exfoliating ingredients such as retinoids, glycolic acid, salicylic acid, and benzoyl peroxide. There's never a season to stop exfoliation, but fall is the time where less is more. Exfoliating gently is also key. To do so, choose natural enzymatic ingredients such as pineapple fruit extract and physical exfoliants that are ground to the texture of fine sand. Skip the exfoliating brushes and devices, and switch to soft facial cloths and sponges such as a konjac facial sponge that is made with 100 percent natural and biodegradable konjac. With a well-designed exfoliant, such as The Spa Dr.'s facial exfoliant, you only need to apply light pressure and your skin should still feel hydrated afterward.

5. **Ensure your sunscreen is broad-spectrum.**

While you have less UVB going into the fall and winter months, UVA levels are still significant skin agers, and they haven't gone anywhere this time of year. Make sure your sunscreen is broad-spectrum or has a high UVA rating. UVB is the wavelength that stimulates vitamin D, so you want more of that this time of year but without the UVA damage.

6. **Use herbal steam.**

With dryer air comes dehydrated skin, so soothing your face with an herbal steam treatment can help your skin feel revitalized and hydrated. Choose fresh seasonal herbs and flowers or dried herbs from late summer, such as calendula and sunflower. If you're feeling tense, add calming essential oils like lavender for mind and skin benefits. The recipes section provides easy DIY essential oil combinations.

If you live in a dryer climate, consider using a humidifier in your bedroom and living areas to support your skin and airways. Find one that allows cool moisture, and be sure to clean it regularly to prevent mold growth. Ideally, choose a humidifier that has an option to add essential oils to get the most bang for your buck.

7. **Pamper yourself with a restorative facial.**

Whether you choose to do this with a natural-product-minded aesthetician or on your own during a spa day at home, you'll enjoy the physical, emotional, and mental benefits of a restorative facial. Start with a relaxing environment and clean, fall-focused skincare. If you're going the DIY route, try to recruit a loved one to join in to boost oxytocin levels from their touch and to fully embrace relaxation. An example of using the DIY skincare fall recipes in this book is to start with the Chia, Honey, and Green Tea Face Wash and then use the Herbal Face Steam along with the Pumpkin Face Mask. After rinsing off the mask, enjoy some relaxation time with soothing music, journaling, and breathwork.

CHAPTER 9

WINTER RESET

(December, January, and February)

What good is the warmth of summer, without the cold of winter to give it sweetness.

—*John Steinbeck*

Winter solstice is the shortest day of the year and is typically around December 20 in the northern hemisphere and around June 20 in the southern hemisphere. For women, winter can be challenging for our hormones, moods, metabolisms, and immune systems. We want to keep our internal fire lit to promote warmth and motivation. I recommend starting the winter 7-Day Natural Beauty Reset as early in the winter as possible to help boost your mood, nutritional status, and hormonal balance. If you followed the fall reset, you're already on the path, and you'll likely find an easy transition. If you're just getting started in winter as your first season, welcome!

A major concern in winter is low vitamin D, which is more common in winter than any other season. Because this vitamin helps regulate certain neurotransmitters, including serotonin, insufficient vitamin D can lead to low mood—so we want to participate in feel-good activities that help combat this effect.[117] In addition, due to changes in our hormones, winter tends to be a time of high set point for metabolism and stress adaptation. As you may recall, thyroid hormone T3 (which helps with metabolism) and cortisol (the stress hormone) are higher in the winter than they are in summer.[118] For that reason, you'll want to modify your food, movement, mindset, and skincare routines to help adjust for these changes. That means focusing more on stress management and mindfulness practices, eating foods and moving in ways that support a healthy metabolism, and choosing soothing and calming skincare.

Leptin sensitivity escalates in the wintertime, while ghrelin levels decrease. This means we tend to feel fuller and less hungry this time of year, keeping our appetite lower during a time when insulin levels tend to be lower. The other positive change is that we have higher melatonin levels in winter compared to summer, so sound sleep should come easier.

Depending upon where you live, winter can bring extremely cold temperatures along with wind, snow, and ice storms. This can be hard on our physical and emotional well-being because it's harder to retreat to nature to restore our moods and bodies. You can't control the weather in winter, but you can change your behavior to boost energy and mood.

Diet-wise, as mentioned in the intro to part II, our average levels of nutrients like folate tend to dip during winter, when

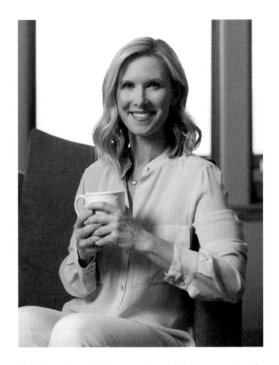

foods rich in folate such as dark-green leafy vegetables are not as abundant.[119] Folate plays a role in serotonin production and adrenal function, so we want to be sure we get extra folate and other foods rich in immune-supportive nutrients. Refer to fall recommendations for other cool-weather nutritional needs.

Winter Food

In many places, little to nothing grows in the winter, so we focus on late fall and early winter harvest as well as produce that was preserved and stored over the growing months. The produce most commonly available in winter includes root vegetables. For the reasons stated in part I (flavor and nutritional value among them), try to resist buying produce that is grown out of season. Selecting seasonal foods has some variability and depends on your location, but there are certain foods that are known to grow better when the sun is closer to the earth and those that grow better when the sun is farther away from the earth, as it is in the winter.

For easier digestion and assimilation, you want to eat more steamed, cooked, and warming foods in the winter than raw, cooling, chilled, or frozen foods. In the list below, I include produce that may not grow where you are but is in season in other places, so the produce is more flavorful and nutritious. For additional seasonal foods, check with your local farmers market to find out which produce is freshest where you live. And remember, choose organic and nongenetically modified as much as possible.

Foods most abundant during winter include:

❄ Grains: Since they store easily in dry, cool locations, enjoy these more seasonal grains throughout the winter.

| BARLEY | QUINOA | WHEAT BERRIES |
| OATS | TRITICALE | |

❄ Fruits: Depending upon your location, you may need to shop outside your area to find fresh produce. Choose these seasonal fruits as close as possible to where you live to ensure freshness and nutritional richness. They typically last longer after being picked than fruit found in spring and summer months.

APPLES	KIWIS	ORANGES
CLEMENTINES	KUMQUATS	PEARS
GOJI BERRIES	LEMONS	PERSIMMONS
GRAPEFRUIT	LIMES	

❊ Vegetables: Root vegetables and heartier vegetables are the focus for winter since they grow in cooler temperatures and last longer after harvest.

BEETS	FRISÉE	POTATOES
BRUSSELS SPROUTS	KALE	RADICCHIO
CABBAGE	LEEKS	RUTABAGAS
CARROTS	MUSHROOMS	SHALLOTS
CAULIFLOWER	OLIVES	SUNCHOKES
CELERY	ONIONS	TURNIPS
ENDIVE	(red, yellow, and white)	WINTER SQUASH
ESCAROLE	PARSNIPS	YAMS

❊ Legumes: Store dried legumes in dry, cool places or use freshly frozen so you can enjoy them through winter months.

BEANS	PEAS
(dried or frozen)	(dried or frozen)

❊ Nuts and seeds: Continue to store nuts and seeds in dry, cool locations to ensure freshness. These are the nuts and seeds you'll find more easily this time of year.

BRAZIL NUTS	CHESTNUTS	PINE NUTS
CASHEWS	HEMP SEEDS	WALNUTS

❄ Animal protein: Meat has seasons too, and these are the ones easiest to find locally and fresh in winter.

BISON	PORK	RABBIT
CANNED ALASKA SALMON	QUAIL	VENISON

❄ Herbs and spices: Enjoy these herbs and spices to keep you warm through the winter months.

BLACK PEPPER	DRIED HERBS	HORSERADISH
CAYENNE	FENNEL	NUTMEG
CHILI PEPPER	GARLIC	PAPRIKA
CINNAMON	GINGER	TURMERIC

❄ Sweets: Comfort foods are often desirable when the sun is farther away, so enjoy these sweeteners for a soul-warming treat.

DATES	MAPLE SYRUP (late winter)	MOLASSES

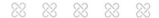

You can also turn to your supply of canned and certain frozen items for additional nourishment and enjoyment.

SAMPLE WINTER MEAL IDEAS FROM RECIPES

Here are a week's worth of ideas to help you get started on the 7-Day Natural Beauty Reset for winter. Feel free to modify, substitute, and repeat recipes throughout. Remember, this is not about restriction or limitations; it's about enjoying the flavors and nourishment available during the season you're in. Make note of which meals you like best so you can continue making them throughout the winter season.

SAMPLE DAY 1

BREAKFAST: Barley Porridge with Pears (page 172)

LUNCH: Warming Venison Stew (page 175)

DINNER: Endive Lentil Salad with Shallot Herb Dressing (page 187)

SNACKS/SWEETS: Nut Crackers with Black Bean Dip (page 188)

SAMPLE DAY 2

BREAKFAST: Beet Ginger Smoothie Juice (page 174)

LUNCH: Barley Salad with Roasted Winter Squash (page 177)

DINNER: Baked Quail with Roasted Parsnips (page 178)

SNACKS/SWEETS: Gluten-Free Gingerbread Muffins (page 189)

SAMPLE DAY 3

BREAKFAST: Persimmon Smoothie Bowl (page 173) topped with Cinnamon Granola (page 173)

LUNCH: Winter Squash Soup (page 184)

TIP: Find ways to maximize your time and minimize prep. For example, make more than the recipe calls for and set aside as leftovers or chop a few days' worth of vegetables and fruit and store in a glass or ceramic container in the refrigerator.

DINNER: Salmon Cabbage Salad (page 186)

SNACKS/SWEETS: Kale Chips (page 171)

SAMPLE DAY 4

BREAKFAST: Make your own oatmeal with gluten-free oats, using cinnamon or maple syrup as your sweetener, and top it with chopped walnuts and late harvest (seasonal) apples or pears

LUNCH: Black Bean and Swiss Chard Soup (page 182)

DINNER: Bison Meatloaf with Garlic Broccoli (page 181)

SNACKS/SWEETS: Baked Apples (page 190)

SAMPLE DAY 5

BREAKFAST: Make your own baked and sliced yams with cinnamon and cashew nut butter

LUNCH: Buy frozen bison patties or use ground bison meat to make your own buffalo burger with a side of winter salad using the Fall Harvest Salad recipe (page 166) for inspiration

DINNER: Leftover Black Bean and Swiss Chard Soup (page 182)

SNACKS/SWEETS: Beau Pa's Cookies (see fall recipe on page 167) using honey instead of maple syrup

SAMPLE DAY 6

BREAKFAST: Make your own smoothie with a combination of one serving of walnuts, cashews, or pine nuts, one serving of seasonal fruit, one serving of endive, escarole, or kale, and 1 cup of cashew milk, hemp milk, or filtered water. Add cinnamon or one to two dates if more sweetness is desired

LUNCH: Potato Leek Soup (page 185)

DINNER: Pork Chops with Leeks and Mashed Yams (page 179)

SNACKS/SWEETS: Carrot Salad (page 190)

SAMPLE DAY 7

BREAKFAST: Persimmon pudding (use the Ginger Chia Pudding with Pomegranate Seeds recipe on page 152 and substitute fruit with persimmons and top with cashews or walnuts)

LUNCH: Make your own kale and apple salad topped with leftover pork chops

DINNER: Leftover Potato Leek Soup (page 185)

SNACKS/SWEETS: Cinnamon Oat Bites (see fall recipe on page 168), using honey instead of maple syrup

❈   ❈   ❈   ❈   ❈

ADDITIONAL SNACK IDEAS FOR WINTER

* Sliced apples with cashew butter
* Fruit salad (any combination of apples, pears, kiwis, oranges, grapefruit, or persimmons)
* Mixed nuts (any combination of walnuts, chestnuts, Brazil nuts, pine nuts, or cashews)
* Celery slices and bean dip
* Sliced pitted dates filled with almond butter
* Kale Chips (see fall recipe on page 171)

Winter Movement

During the winter, we may feel less motivated to exercise due to hormonal changes and less sunlight. While we may feel more inclined to catch up on sleep, that doesn't mean we rest all winter. As always, it's about finding balance. Winter isn't the best time to start something new that requires a lot of our energy, so don't beat yourself up if you don't possess your usual level of motivation. You can also take the time to rest and reflect and make plans to fit in your exercise routine the following day.

Recommendations during this season include stretching and yoga postures that will help rekindle our motivation for movement. We aren't hibernating like the bears and life as a modern woman doesn't slow down, so we'll want to keep exercising to support our energy, mood, metabolism, and sleep through winter. I'll also share how to make a simple home gym with some resistance bands and a chair.

Enjoying the great outdoors in winter months is all about the gear. I've lived in just about every area of the United States and am familiar with winters in all zones and have all kinds of weather-appropriate gear. Layers and comfort are key for winter movement.

Start with a thin layer of wool or synthetic material so that when you sweat, it won't make you cold. Follow that with a temperature-appropriate layer such as a medium-weight wool or synthetic material and a shell or a waterproof or windproof outer layer. Avoid cotton as it absorbs moisture and will leave you feeling cold. Don't forget a hat and gloves plus appropriate shoes with wool or synthetic socks. You want to increase circulation and make sure you don't get chilled. You may want to also wear a neck or face covering in wintry weather if there is wind, freezing temperatures, or precipitation.

Listen to your body and take it easy if and when your muscles and joints feel achy, but don't be afraid to challenge yourself physically to increase circulation and give your mood a boost. Movement is essential during the winter, even when it doesn't always feel easy to get motivated. Look to friends and your community (classes) to help motivate you, but, again, don't be hard on yourself if you take a day off. Going more than a day without movement, though, may impact your sense of well-being, so do your best to at least bundle up and get outdoors for a walk around the block.

Setting yourself up for success is key during winter months. Allow for time and plan ahead to reduce stress and allow movement to be seamless.

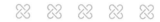

7 Movements for Winter

1. **Find an exercise partner and head to the gym.**
   Setting a date with a fitness friend can give you that extra motivation you need to move your body. When working out with a friend, plan on more time for your workout. Instead of thirty minutes, allow for forty-five minutes to an hour so you have time to socialize. This way, you'll alleviate stress and build those social connections so many of us crave in the wintertime. Opt for a workout that activates a variety of muscle groups. If you and your workout buddy are new to exercise, sign up for a group fitness class or hire a personal trainer for an hour to create a plan together. Use an old-school journal to record your fitness goals and milestones by hand, or tap into the benefits of an app to track your progress virtually. Doing so will help you stay motivated to keep sweating it out!

2. **Sign up for an online video class for a stretch and flex.**
   You may not feel motivated to leave your home and embrace the winter elements, so doing an online or app-based workout gives you no excuse to skip your daily movement practice. From fitness level to type of platform (online or in person), there's no shortage of options out there! If you aren't

sure where to start, consult a friend or a personal trainer for advice. If you're going to take a class, I recommend signing up for a live paid-for option rather than a free prerecorded one because this way you're more likely to stay committed. Again, it's about setting yourself up for success. Choose a stretching class if your muscles are feeling stiff or if you're feeling unmotivated. Choose a strengthening class when you want to ramp up your energy level and are ready for some muscle-building fun. Go at your own pace and speed. Above all, avoid the temptation to get fit in a day. Take it slow to avoid injury, and build a routine you can sustain for the season and beyond.

3. **Go for a brisk walk, bike, or run during your lunch break.**
   As long as you can squeeze in a meal before or after, try to fit fitness into your lunch break. It's a great opportunity to step away from your desk and take a breath of fresh air! If you're going hard, eat afterward; if you're taking only a stroll, eat beforehand. Just be sure to be mindful of portions if you're exercising after eating. If lunchtime doesn't work, find another time and add it to your calendar as you would any other commitment.

   Because you'll be heading outdoors, don't forget your gear! Nab good-quality shoes with traction if it's snowy or icy, and remember your layers as well as head and hand protection. If there's wind, start your workout in the direction facing the wind. This way, when you're at your sweatiest, you'll have your back to the wind and the hardest part will be over.

4. **Do a morning workout.**
   Wake up and put your workout clothes on before you get sidetracked by anything else. Here's a simple workout with a chair and resistance bands. Simply do each of these exercises for thirty to sixty seconds, rest for a minute, and then repeat for three total rounds.

   ❊ Booty burn: Position your body facedown with your elbows and knees on the floor. You can use a yoga mat or towel to protect your hands and knees from a hard floor. Lift your right leg toward the ceiling, keeping your leg bent and your foot flexed. Lift until you feel the burn in your glute and then lower your leg to the ground. Repeat with the same leg for thirty seconds and then switch to the left leg.

   ❊ Lateral walk: You'll need a resistance band for this one. Keeping the band flat, wrap it around both legs just above each ankle. Start with your feet shoulder-width apart with the band taut. Bend your knees slightly and move into a half-squat position.

Keep your feet in line with your shoulders and your back straight. Stay low with your hips level, take a step sideways with your right leg, and move in and out to the right for ten repetitions. Switch legs to do another ten sidesteps on the left side.

* Classic plank: Place your forearms on the floor with elbows aligned below your shoulders and arms parallel to your body. Orient your body horizontally, and press your toes into the floor, squeezing your glutes to stabilize your body. Be careful not to lock or hyperextend your knees. Keep your neck and spine straight as you look down at the floor. Hold for twenty to sixty seconds, and remember to breathe!

* High knees or running in place: For thirty to sixty seconds, stand up straight and either march or run in place. Try to lift your knees high, at or above the level of your waistline, if possible, being mindful not to strain your back.

* Assisted squats: You'll need a chair or bench for this one. Bend your knees at a 90-degree angle a couple of inches in front of your chair. Lower your butt slowly, not quite reaching the seat, and then stand up with a slight pelvic tilt forward to fully engage the glute muscles as you straighten your legs. Repeat for thirty to sixty seconds.

5. **Find a winter-friendly activity.**
   Embrace the season! Rent, buy, borrow, or grab your gear and go! Ski, snowshoe, skate, ski, ice skate, sled, or just walk or run around the neighborhood. You can even shovel snow if it's falling in your area to get a workout in during chore time. If it doesn't snow where you live, consider finding some so you can participate in a cold-weather activity. If you're not used to higher altitudes, give yourself time to adjust. Don't skimp on water—cold temperatures can be just as dehydrating as hot ones. Ease into these activities, especially if they're new for you. Take time to warm up and stretch. And don't forget your mineral-based sunscreen for exposed skin because the snow reflects and intensifies sun exposure. If it's early or late in the day, enjoy ten minutes of sun exposure for a quick vitamin D boost before applying your sunscreen.

6. **Take a yoga class.**
   Yoga comes in many forms and styles. Teachers vary in abilities and techniques, so choose your class and teacher wisely. For winter, you want to focus on improving circulation while being mindful that your muscles and joints may be feeling stiff, and your mind may be more interested in relaxation. Hot yoga can be a nice option to help warm up the body and ease your way into yoga poses. One option

is Bikram, where the room temperature is usually around 105 degrees Fahrenheit. Talk with your healthcare provider if you're pregnant or have an existing health issue such as heart disease or a history of heat stroke before doing a hot yoga class.

Like everything, though, it's about balance. In the wintertime, your adrenals will already be stressed—and pushing yourself too hard physically will make them even more so. Instead, take it easy as you choose your yoga location, temperature, and poses. Also, be sure to drink extra water with electrolytes if you're doing hot yoga, especially in the winter when the air is already dryer and you have a greater chance of dehydration.

Here are a few of my wintertime favorite yoga poses to find online or ask for in your local yoga class. I like these because they're gentle yet help stoke our internal fire. Consider holding these poses a bit longer than usual to challenge yourself and connect more deeply. And don't forget to breathe!

- ❄ Butterfly pose
- ❄ Side-lying twist
- ❄ Seated forward bend
- ❄ Locust pose
- ❄ Legs up the wall
- ❄ Savasana

7. **Try a new fitness class or sport and seek out fun.**

Get those feel-good hormones pumping to lift your wintertime mood! There are so many activities that can help you do just that: spinning, rock climbing, dance, Pilates, or kickboxing classes, and indoor tennis or pickleball. Try one that sounds fun, and grabbing a friend or family member to join you may help reduce the fear of trying something new. If the activity doesn't strike your fancy, experiment and try a different one.

You're more likely to overcome the resistance to workouts if you're inspired and looking forward to them. It may take time and a sense of adventure, but trying something new stimulates positive changes for your brain, especially as you age.[120] It helps your brain's neuroplasticity, which is how well your brain is able to adapt.

Winter Mindset

Winter is the season to rest and restore. It is an ideal time for mindset practices such as forgiveness exercises, gratitude journaling, and deeper, longer meditations. These approaches will help you gain a greater awareness of your mood and needs, which will shift through the season. You may feel more sluggish this time of year due to elevated melatonin levels, but avoid napping for more than fifteen minutes during the day because more than a short power nap can make it harder to fall asleep at night. That said, if your body is craving an extra hour of sleep, give yourself permission to take that extra time to recharge. Ample z's are crucial for your body to reset.

7 Mindset Activities for Winter

1. **Start your mornings with invigorating breathwork and yoga.**
   Full yogic breathing is known for its revitalizing effects and helps alleviate stress and stimulate circulation around the vital organs. Do this exercise before breakfast on an empty stomach for five to fifteen minutes with your eyes closed. You may want to set a timer so you don't have to open your eyes to check the time.

   Start in a comfortable position, either seated with your spine straight or lying on your back. Close your eyes, find a still place in your mind, and allow your thoughts to quiet. Relax your body. Bring your attention to your breathing and inhale deeply, slowly allowing your breath to fill your lower abdomen toward your navel and away from your spine. Once that area is filled, continue your inhalation to your mid-torso, continuing to draw your breath upward from your navel to your ribs, and gently expand your diaphragm as your breath continues to rise. Carry your breath to your upper chest into the area of your heart, sternum, and then into your shoulders and the lower part

of your neck. Pause for a moment at the top of the inhalation. Then allow for a long, slow exhalation, reversing the flow of your breath through the path it traveled upward. Specifically, relax your body beginning at your upper chest while dropping your breath down and in toward your spine. Move your awareness to your mid-torso, noticing your ribs and navel pull in toward your spine. Finally, continue your exhale from the lower abdomen, feeling this space draw inward toward your spine. Take a moment to pause before repeating your next breathing cycle, starting with your inhalation. After you've completed several rounds of this exercise, allow your breathing pattern to return to normal before opening your eyes and going about your day.

2. **Window bathe in the morning**
   Wintertime often causes a drop in mood, but it doesn't have to. Feel more cheerful without having to brave the elements by basking in the sunlight shining through a window in your home or workplace for five to twenty minutes. While most windows block the UVB rays your body needs to make vitamin D, you can still reap some benefits. Exposure to sunlight is known for its ability to stimulate serotonin release, which happens when our eyes (retina) and skin come in contact with the sun's rays.[121] The

benefits appear with UVA exposure, too.[122] It's best to do this on a day when the sun is shining brightly, but be mindful that the UVA rays coming through the window can still be damaging to your skin, so choose your location as well as time of day wisely. Window bathing is not as refreshing as breathing in the fresh air in direct sunlight, nor will it allow for beneficial vitamin D synthesis in the skin, so I encourage you to still bundle up and get outdoors for some vitamin D and fresh air.

3. **Cozy up by the fire with a great book and a cup of warming tea.**
    If you live in a cooler climate, you can warm your body and soul with some fireside time. If you don't have a gas or wood-burning stove, curl up in a lounge chair or sofa with a cozy blanket. Sipping tea is a nice addition, especially drinking one with warming spices like ginger, cinnamon, cardamom, and cloves. You can choose to make your own tea or pick some up at your local grocery, health, or specialty food store. If you have a furry friend or a loving companion, ask them to join you to bump up your oxytocin.

4. **Engage with your community to combat loneliness.**
    In the winter, we may feel more isolated and alone compared to other times of the year. A review of thirty studies on loneliness and social isolation showed an increase in system inflammation,[123] and other research has unveiled a negative impact on brain chemistry and function from prolonged isolation.[124] Take proactive steps to feel less alone this time of year. For instance, attend group classes and schedule meetups with friends. Identify people with similar interests to form new social bonds. Consider joining a book club or a religious studies group. If you enjoy meditation or yoga, search for classes in your area where you can make new friends or go with ones you already have. If you're managing the effects of trauma from a previous life event, consider joining a support group to connect with your peers. Be sure to choose a group with a guide or coach who has reached the other side of recovery to help ensure the experience is a positive one for you. The goal is to help you feel supported and less alone—essentially, to feel that you are part of a community on which you can lean.

TIP: Keep a daily journal and write about your activities and insights.

5. **Give your oxytocin a boost with touch.**
   Snuggle up with a pet, get a massage or facial, hug a friend, or make love with your partner. All of these activities are known to elevate our oxytocin, which helps us feel more connected, appreciated, and loved. Don't have a partner or pet? Treat yourself to a massage. This time of year, we're more likely to experience muscle tightness and joint stiffness. Get a foam roller, a tennis ball, or a lacrosse ball and work out sore muscles. Alternatively, use sesame or almond oil with a few drops of sweet orange or rose essential oil and give yourself a foot or scalp massage. Have a partner or friend? Have them join in.

6. **Laugh.**
   Read a funny book, tell jokes, listen to a humorous podcast, or watch a silly movie. This may seem like a simple exercise, but it's essential this time of year. Laughter helps decrease cortisol and alter dopamine and serotonin activity.[125] It has been shown to boost our immunity, improve our social bonding,[126] decrease pain,[127] and instantly shift us to a more positive mood. And it's free and easy! You can laugh alone or find humor with a friend. Look online for three funny jokes and call a friend today to share them. See how you both respond, and don't forget to journal about it.

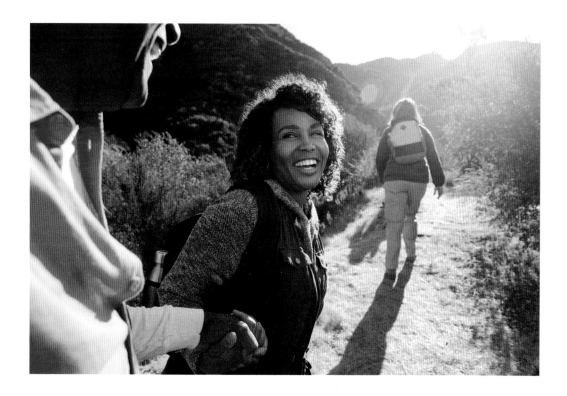

How do you feel physically and emotionally after laughing?

7. **Create a bedtime ritual.**
As mentioned in chapter 4, sleep is essential for hormonal balance and to support overall well-being. Because darkness is on our side in winter, it's the perfect time to establish an effective bedtime ritual. Personalize yours to your taste. At least an hour before bed, turn off electronics, dim the lights, light a candle, listen to soothing music, read a relaxing paperback or hardcover book (avoid e-readers), stretch, enjoy some calming breathwork, pray, meditate, pamper with soothing skincare, breathe in some de-stressing essentials oil, or take a bath with muscle-easing bath salts. Here is a recipe for a soothing bath:

Body Bath Salts

INGREDIENTS:

- 2 cups Epsom salt
- ½ cup baking soda
- 1 cup Himalayan crystal salt
- 30 to 40 drops of lavender essential oils

Combine the ingredients in a glass, ceramic, or metal container. Add to warm bath and soak for 15 to 20 minutes.

Winter Skincare

With the sun farther away and our spending more time indoors, our skin can appear dry and dull, so the focus of winter skincare is hydration and nourishment. Extra time indoors with artificial heat from forced air or radiant heat means your skin may be even drier this time of year. DIY options include the Winter Body Scrub, Cleansing Body Oil, and Soothing Lip Balm (see recipes).

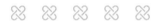

7 Skincare Practices for Winter

1. **Use a layer of cleansing oil on skin before getting in a warm shower.**
When the weather is cold, we're tempted to shower with extra-hot water to warm our bodies, but the problem is that hot water evaporates quickly and dries out skin. During this time of year, I encourage you to minimize superhot showers. And before stepping in the shower or bath, apply a cleansing oil to your skin to help hydrate and protect it.

   Follow the Cleansing Body Oil recipe. Apply 1 to 2 tablespoons to your entire body and then step into a warm shower or bath. Allow this oil to be your cleanser instead of a bar of soap, which has a high pH and strips the skin of natural oils. When you're finished bathing, pat your skin rather than rub it dry so you don't remove all of those fabulous oils on your skin. Be sure to avoid skincare products containing alcohol and those with a high pH, such as the typical bar of soap, which is going to have a pH over 5.4.

2. **Use natural lip moisturizers.**
   Don't forget your lips! They need extra TLC during the winter months because chapping is common when we're braving the elements. Before you slather on the lip gloss, ChapStick, or lip balm, study the ingredients list. Most lip products contain potentially toxic ingredients such as fragrance, petrolatum, and mineral oil. What you put on your lips ends up inside your body even more so than skincare products applied to other parts of your body. When you lick your lips, or drink a beverage or eat food, much of what's on your lips ends up in your mouth. This means lip-care products are one of the most important products to be toxic-free. You can make a lip balm (see the recipe for Soothing Lip Balm) or buy one made with natural ingredients such as coconut oil, shea butter, vitamin E, beeswax, and organic essential oils.

3. **Steam your face with a hydrating mask or cleanser.**
   A facial steam (see Herbal Face Steam recipe on page 226) can feel great this time of year, but be mindful that hot water can further dry out your skin. So apply a soothing natural face mask or cleanser to your skin before doing a face steam. I recommend applying the Pumpkin Face Mask (see fall recipe on page 227) or a natural skincare routine such as applying The Spa Dr.'s Step 1 Gentle Cleanser to your face and then doing an herbal face steam with dried herbs such as rose petals and rose essential oil.

4. **Increase your hydration habit, especially at night.**
   As you can tell from the previous three skincare practices, hydration is key for winter. Because it's easier to catch up on your sleep in winter months compared to the other seasons of the year, it's also a great time to focus on hydrating your skin as you sleep. For your evening skincare routine, start with a creamy oil-based cleanser. The cooler winter air offers a skin perk. Compared to the other seasons, our pores are smaller and less likely to get clogged, so don't be afraid to use plant-based oils, even if you have acne-prone skin. Your skin should not feel tight after cleansing if you're using the right cleanser. Follow with an antioxidant serum, such as The Spa Dr.'s Step 2 Antioxidant Serum; a moisturizer, such as The Spa Dr.'s Step 3 Enriched Moisturizer; and finish your routine by doing a self-massage with face oil. Choose a natural face oil such as The Spa Dr.'s Step 4 Glow Boost or make a blend with your favorite plant-based oils according to your skin

type and needs. For example, jojoba oil is typically great for oilier skin and almond oil works well for drier skin types. Place the application of oil in your palms and warm it by rubbing your hands together and then pressing it into your skin (to improve absorption), focusing on the drier skin areas.

5. **Exfoliate dry skin.**
Done correctly, exfoliation helps remove dead, dull surface skin cells to reveal the fresh, glowing skin underneath. It also helps detox skin and enhance the effectiveness of your daily skincare routine by increasing absorption of products. There are numerous exfoliants, but only two main types: physical and chemical.

Chemical exfoliants, including alpha hydroxy acids (AHAs) such as glycolic acid and beta hydroxy acids (BHAs) such as salicylic acid, have enzymatic properties that help slough off dead skin cells. Physical exfoliants are those that contain a scrub-type ingredient that causes the exfoliation, such as sugar or coffee grounds. Both chemical and physical exfoliants have their place, but we want to be careful not to over exfoliate with either harsh chemical or physical exfoliants, thereby damaging the skin's microbiome and barrier function.

When using chemical exfoliants, start with more natural versions like papaya or pineapple fruit extract. If you use products with synthetic ingredients, use as directed on the bottle or follow the advice of a well-trained aesthetician. Avoid exfoliants with coarsely ground ingredients and brushes because they may cause microscopic tears that damage the skin. The Spa Dr.'s exfoliant uses finely ground cultured freshwater pearls to create a gentle yet effective physical exfoliation.

Here are a few of my favorite exfoliant ingredients for DIY skincare:

❋ Papaya: A rich source of vitamins A, C, and E; contains the papain enzyme, which is a natural exfoliant.
❋ Pomegranate seeds: Grind these in a blender until smooth for an antioxidant-rich exfoliant.
❋ Yogurt: The lactic acid in yogurt is a natural exfoliant; it helps balance the skin's pH.

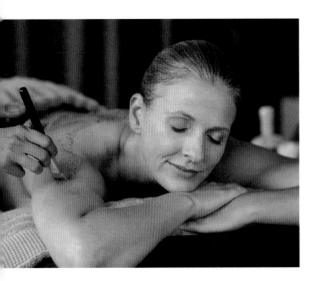

Whether you're making your own exfoliant or looking to purchase one made with natural and organic ingredients, don't miss this step in your skincare routine. Spend extra time on rough spots such as knees, elbows, heels, and ankles. To make your own body exfoliant, see the recipe for Winter Body Scrub.

Although exfoliation offers plenty of benefits, it can also harm your skin if you don't follow best practices. Avoid or minimize exfoliating during the following circumstances:

- If you plan to be in direct sunlight for an extended period of time
- If you have extremely sensitive skin
- If you're using a dermatology prescription such as topical steroids, antibiotics, Retin-A, or Accutane
- If your skin is broken, inflamed, sunburned, or otherwise damaged
- If you have been swimming or hot tubbing in chlorinated water
- If your face is windburned, such as after a day of skiing

Facial exfoliants should be much gentler than body exfoliants because the skin on your face is more delicate.

6. **Consider a procedure to address your skin's unique needs.**
Now is the best time for minimally invasive procedures you may consider that typically have more potential for sensitivity to sun and damage. Here are three examples of in-office procedures that are less invasive than plastic surgery and do not include any injections of potentially toxic ingredients:

a. **Microneedling.** A roughly fifteen-minute in-office procedure, microneedling involves making tiny needle punctures in the top layer of skin with the goal of improving the skin's overall texture and appearance. The needles are energized with radio frequency to help stimulate collagen growth in the skin. The procedure is relatively low cost, only mildly painful, and it doesn't involve the injection of artificial ingredients. A growing number of dermatologists, plastic surgeons, and integrative doctors are performing these procedures in their offices because of their benefits and the minimal recovery time involved.

b. **Platelet-rich plasma (PRP) facials.** Sometimes called vampire facials, PRP facials can give microneedling a boost. During the microneedling process, the skin opens up and can more readily absorb products. In this case, PRP appears to reach the inner layers of skin, where it aids in the regeneration process. PRP facials involve injecting your own platelets and fibrin, which is obtained from your blood, with the aim of reducing wrinkles and scars in the face, hands, and neck. It also appears to support stem cell proliferation and new collagen formation.[128] Patients whom I've referred for this treatment have noticed a visible reduction in fine lines and wrinkles as well as less acne scarring after three treatments.

c.   **Cosmetic lasers.** This procedure can help tighten the skin, promoting smoothness and reducing the appearance of brown spots. As with any procedure, using lasers to correct skin issues poses certain risks, such as equipment malfunction and user error. While they can yield results and don't involve the use of toxic chemicals, certain lasers are more safe and effective than others.

If you're looking for a completely natural look without the help of technology, you may choose to skip these types of procedures. It's all about making educated and healthy decisions that support your short- and long-term goals.

Because these types of treatment can make your skin more sensitive to sun damage, please don't forget your sunscreen! While you have less UVB in the winter, remember that UVA levels are skin agers. Make sure your sunscreen is broad-spectrum or has a high UVA rating.

7.   **Get a winter facial.**
Whether you choose to pamper yourself with a DIY spa day or one outside of the home, take time for this self-care. Having a spa day or hour can help reduce cortisol, boost oxytocin, and give you a moment to reset. Because you're likely spending less time in the sun, now is the time to consider more exfoliating treatments. Look to seasonal ingredients such as citrus, persimmons, and oats if you're going the DIY route. For store-bought products, check the labels to ensure they don't contain potentially toxic ingredients, or ask your spa of choice about the quality and contents of their products.

CHAPTER 10

SPRING RESET

(March, April, and May)

Spring is nature's way of saying, "Let's party!"

—Robin Williams

Spring equinox is when our planet starts to tilt more in the sun's direction and is a great time to start the spring 7-Day Natural Beauty Reset. It's important to follow the sun in the area you live to restore harmony within your body. For those of you who live in the northern hemisphere, the spring equinox is on the 19th, 20th, or 21st, depending upon the year, in March, and for those in the southern hemisphere, it is in September. If that exact date doesn't work for you to dive into your reset, anytime in spring works beautifully.

The equinox is when the day and night are of nearly equal length. The spring equinox is a time of buds bursting and leaves unfolding. Many animals, insects, and plants are waking from their winter slumber. Worms are appearing in the soil; birds are migrating north, following the path of the sun; daffodils are breaking through; and fresh produce is becoming more readily available for our nourishment. For us humans, it's time to lighten up and shed our winter coat. In winter our digestion typically slows and our stress response may be a bit more challenged, so ease your way into the early spring by supporting your digestive tract and adrenals with dietary, exercise, and mindset shifts.

If you're considering starting or adding to your family, spring is the perfect time for reproduction and growth. Exposure to more sunshine increases our production of follicle-stimulating hormone, which helps stimulate ovulation. Even if fertility goals are not in your current forecast, spring is a great time to rebalance hormones, revitalize, and shake off the winter blues. We're shifting from high-cortisol times of winter to low-cortisol summers, and our estrogen levels are increasing as we approach summer.

Spring Food

Spring is the perfect time to cleanse your body and cut out substances that challenge your liver such as sugar, processed foods, alcohol, and caffeine. In spring, it's best to keep your meals simple and clean with less focus on fruits and grains, because they're not as readily available as they are at other times of year, and more focus on sprouts, greens, and spring protein, which are easier to find fresh and local, giving you a nutritional boost for your natural beauty.

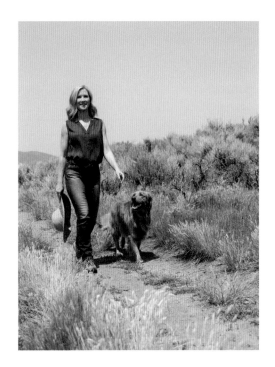

To eat within season, start weaning yourself off eating cold-weather produce like winter squash and root veggies. Eating light rather than heavy meals is key to resetting your metabolism and hormones. In early spring, if your environment still has cooler weather, the majority of your meals will ideally be at least lightly cooked or steamed so your body is not chilled, and your digestion is not stressed.

Bitter greens like mustard greens help stimulate digestion after the sluggish winter months. In the legumes department, focus on options that are easier to digest such as snow and snap peas. If you like going grain-free, now is the time of year to axe grains from your diet. On the other hand, if you want to consume grains, choose light options like quinoa, amaranth, and millet. As the temperature warms up, enjoy fresh, hydrating juices and more raw produce. Foods to avoid or minimize in spring are cucumbers, bananas, pineapples, melons, dates, coconuts, beef, and pork.

During spring, focus on mostly grain-free meals, and those eating meat will include chicken, eggs, and certain types of fish and shellfish. The foods found most abundantly in nature during spring are the ones most nourishing and restorative for our bodies and hormones. For additional seasonal foods, check with your local farmers market to find out which produce is freshest where you live. And remember, choose organic and nongenetically modified as much as possible.

Foods most abundant during spring include:

❅ Fruits: After the cooler temperatures of winter, there may be limited fresh fruit in your area. Look for spring crops like strawberries and then look for seasonal produce shipped to your area from warmer climates.

APRICOTS	GRAPEFRUIT	LEMONS
(late spring)	GUAVA	LYCHEE
CHERRIES	JACKFRUIT	STRAWBERRIES
(late spring)	KUMQUATS	

❅ Vegetables: Spring is the time of renewal and beginnings, so focus your vegetables on sprouts, spring greens, new potatoes, and other seasonal produce.

ARTICHOKES	GREEN-LEAF	RHUBARB
ARUGULA	SPROUTS	(late spring)
ASPARAGUS	MICROGREENS	SPRING GREENS
CABBAGES	MOREL MUSHROOMS	(arugula, dandelion greens,
COLLARD GREENS	MUSTARD GREENS	pea shoots, and watercress)
DANDELIONS	NEW POTATOES	SPRING ONIONS
FIDDLEHEADS	RADISHES	

❅ Legumes: Now is the time to switch from dried and frozen to fresh seasonal legumes.

FAVA BEANS	PEAS
	(garden, snap, snow, etc.)

❊ Nuts and seeds: These nuts are easier to find fresh in spring and provide essential fatty acids to help nourish your body after winter.

CASHEWS   MACADAMIA NUTS   WALNUTS

❊ Animal protein: Chickens and eggs are a sign of spring, making it the perfect time to enjoy these in your meals along with sardines and shellfish.

CHICKENS   SARDINES
EGGS   SHELLFISH

❊ Herbs and spices: Enjoy the fresh flavors of spring with these seasonal herbs.

CHIVES   DILL   GREEN GARLIC
CILANTRO   GARLIC SCAPES   MINT
                                    PARSLEY

❊ Sweets: Spring is a good time to lay off the sweets to cleanse and renew. If you need the occasional sweet, enjoy a bit of seasonal maple syrup.

MAPLE SYRUP

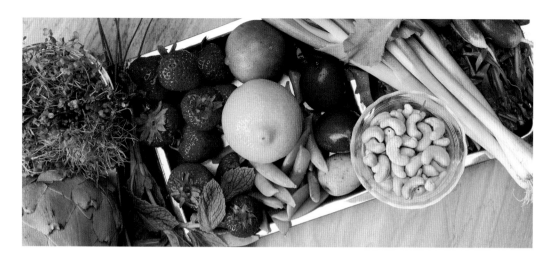

SAMPLE SPRING MEAL IDEAS FROM RECIPES

Here are a week's worth of ideas to help you get started on the 7-Day Natural Beauty Reset for spring. Feel free to modify, substitute, and repeat recipes throughout. Remember, this is not about restriction or limitations; it's about enjoying the flavors and nourishment available during the season you're in. Make note of the spring meals your body and mind enjoy the most so you can enjoy them throughout the spring season.

SAMPLE DAY 1

BREAKFAST: Poached Eggs over Arugula and Sprouts Bowl (page 192)

LUNCH: Spring Greens and Strawberry Salad (page 199)

DINNER: Spring Chive Soup (page 196)

SNACKS/SWEETS: Cherry Chocolate Mousse (page 207)

TIP: Find ways to maximize your time and minimize prep. For example, make more than a recipe calls for and set aside as leftovers or chop a few days' worth of vegetables and fruit and store in a glass or ceramic container in the refrigerator.

SAMPLE DAY 2

BREAKFAST: Spring Greens Smoothie (page 191)

LUNCH: Braised Turnips and Greens Bowl (page 201)

DINNER: Pacific Sardines Salad (page 196)

SNACKS/SWEETS: Macadamia Nut Custard (page 204)

SAMPLE DAY 3

BREAKFAST: Dandelion Strawberry Bowl with Macadamia Nuts (page 194)

LUNCH: Creamy Cilantro Green Pea Soup (page 197)

DINNER: Pan Seared Scallops over Collard Greens (page 194)

SNACKS/SWEETS: Spring Onion Hummus with Nut Crackers (page 208)

SAMPLE DAY 4

BREAKFAST: Make your own breakfast bowl with 1 cup of spring greens, 1 cup of seasonal fruit, and one serving of nuts or two poached eggs

LUNCH: Creamy Artichoke Soup (page 203)

DINNER: Free-Range Spring Apricot Chicken with Leeks (page 202)

SNACKS/SWEETS: Strawberry Rhubarb Crisp (page 206)

SAMPLE DAY 5

BREAKFAST: Make your own smoothie with one serving of spring greens, 1 cup of unsweetened macadamia or cashew milk, one serving of macadamia nuts, and one serving of seasonal fruit

LUNCH: Leftover Free-Range Spring Apricot Chicken with Leeks

DINNER: Make your own seasonal salad with spring greens and an oil, vinegar, and spring herbs dressing and top it with shrimp

SNACKS/SWEETS: Make your own potato salad using new potatoes and avocado mayonnaise

SAMPLE DAY 6

BREAKFAST: Kiwi Mint Smoothie with Bee Pollen (page 191)

LUNCH: Chicken with Watercress Wraps (page 202)

DINNER: Asparagus and Fava Bean Salad (page 198)

SNACKS/SWEETS: Egg Dip with Veggies (page 204)

SAMPLE DAY 7

BREAKFAST: Make your own smoothie with one serving of spring greens, 1 cup of unsweetened macadamia or cashew milk, one serving of macadamia nuts, and one serving of seasonal fruit

LUNCH: Combine leftover chicken salad from the Chicken with Watercress Wraps with chopped seasonal vegetables and a drizzle of olive oil

DINNER: Make your own Caesar salad using Romaine lettuce and store-bought gluten-free croutons and Caesar dressing

SNACKS/SWEETS: Sardines with Nut Crackers (page 188)

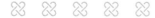

ADDITIONAL SNACK IDEAS FOR SPRING

- Seasonal mixed fruit (any combination of kumquats, strawberries, jackfruit, lychee, apricots [late spring], cherries [late spring], grapefruit, or guava)
- Mixed nuts (any combination of walnuts, cashews, or macadamia nuts)
- Mint tea
- Shrimp with cocktail sauce
- Steamed artichoke with avocado mayonnaise dip
- Deviled eggs

Spring Movement

Spring is a time of getting back outdoors on a more regular basis to ground yourself and reconnect with nature. As you know by now, studies have shown that time in nature where people feel safe is an effective way to manage stress.[129] It lowers blood pressure and stress hormones, supports immune system function, improves mood, increases self-esteem, and reduces anxiety. Take your movement to the outdoors for more than a few potential perks!

One of the reasons immersing ourselves in nature is so healing has to do with dirt and microorganisms.[130] Interestingly, the soil and our digestive tract contain about the same number of active microorganisms, and yet our gut microbiota diversity is only about 10 percent of the soil's biodiversity, making nature a bit wiser. Unfortunately, human microbiota diversity has greatly decreased with our transition from hunter-gatherer to an urbanized society. So it's essential for us to do our best to get back to nature to help support our biodiversity, especially after a long winter indoors.

Different types of physical activity influence our hormonal balance. For example, during resistance exercise, testosterone production can be triggered in healthy women.[131] High-intensity workouts with heavy weights can stimulate the production of human growth hormone.[132] And low-intensity exercise can decrease our stress hormone cortisol, while high-intensity exercise tends to increase cortisol.[133]

With this in mind, and remembering that our hormones are a motivation factor when it comes to exercise, I will recommend movement modifications to jumpstart the spring reset. Because spring is the time of "waking up," recommended exercises during these seven days are relatively more restorative with a focus on certain types of yoga, stretching, and walks in nature. I encourage you to exercise in the morning with the early rise of the sun to help your body wake up with a healthy dose of morning cortisol.

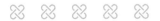

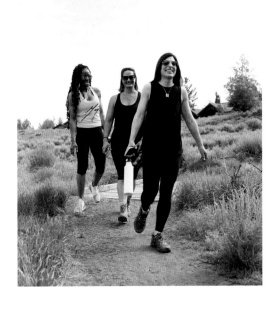

7 Movements for Spring

1. **Take a quiet sunrise hike.**

    Set your alarm because awakening with the changing time of sunrise may not initially feel intuitive, but it will help you get off on the right foot for a spring reset. Turn your hike into a meditation by focusing on the sights, scents, and sounds around you. If thoughts of your pending to-do list drift in, acknowledge them briefly and then return your focus to your senses and the rising sun while you take each step. If you only have time for a twenty-minute hike, take it! If you have time for an hour or two, that's great, too. The key is finding time and making it happen.

2. **Enjoy chest-opening yoga poses.**
    Opening up your body and mind to allow for more vitality in your life is a great focus for spring. Practice yoga poses that open tight areas such as the chest and help wake up your body from the colder and more sedentary months behind you.

    Some yoga poses to try with your yoga teacher or to learn how to do in an online class include the following poses and will help bring your body back to life and bloom into spring. Backbends help bring more energy into the chest, and standing poses will help activate and ground you.

    - Sun salutation
    - Cobra pose
    - Fish pose
    - Camel pose
    - Lunge prayer twist
    - Savasana

    As with all yoga and exercise, be sure to use proper form, and if you're new to these exercises, ease your way in rather than try to turn into a yogi in a day.

3. **Take an afternoon brisk walk, hike, or run in your nearby park or forest.**
    Instead of taking a nap, beat afternoon fatigue by putting on your running shoes and getting outdoors. You'll likely be revitalized by the crisp air, recent rain, or breeze on your skin. If you still need that ten-minute snooze, you can take it, but getting the exercise in first will help you determine whether you're truly sleep deprived or just in need of some fresh air and improved circulation. Spring weather can be unpredictable, so set yourself up for success by having a light rain jacket handy and shoes with good tread and support.

4. **Get in a morning workout.**
    Spring is about waking up, so push yourself a bit to reset your clock by waking up forty-five minutes earlier than usual to fit in an AM workout. Plan ahead with an earlier bedtime so you're not starting off your day with

sleep deprivation, which will only further stress your adrenals. If you're not typically a morning person, start slow. For example, try a twenty-minute cycle of simple side steps, squats, and lunges. Then if you're ready to step it up, add in another ten to fifteen minutes and find some stairs to walk (or run) up and down on or do some chair squats. Add in some upper-body strengthening with push-ups or planks.

5. **Stretch and reflect.**
As women, we often try to do it all and push ourselves to the point of exhaustion. But resist this urge and listen to your body. When you need to rest, rest. When you have the energy to push yourself, push yourself. But if you burn yourself out mentally and physically, you will only set yourself back, losing motivation and potentially injuring yourself.

If you're noticing that your body is tense and you're ruminating rather than relaxing, it's time to stretch and reflect. First sit quietly and check in with your body. Where do you feel tension? Do you have pain, aches, spasms, or other physical discomforts? Taking mental notes can help you determine which muscle groups to focus on. If you have extreme pain from a suspected injury, touch base with your healthcare provider for treatment. If your body is simply tight or tense but not due to an

injury or strain, go ahead with stretches that address those areas. Common areas of muscle tension include the back of the upper legs, the calves, the sides of the upper legs, the lower back, and the sides of the neck. Be gentle as you stretch and reflect on how your body responds.

6. **Jump into a more intense workout.**
After you've rested sufficiently, step up the intensity and duration of your movement. Speed up your walk to a power walk, go from a brisk walk to a jog, or take your flat hike to one with more hilly terrain. Increase the duration if you can: if you normally exercise for twenty minutes, try bumping it up to thirty minutes or from thirty to forty-five minutes, for instance. Pay attention to how your body responds, and remember not to overdo it.

If you're already an athlete, today might be more about slowing down and doing the opposite of an intense workout. The idea is to mix up your routine today and spring forward into something different.

Don't forget to stay hydrated with water and consume electrolytes. Wear appropriate shoes and outdoor gear. Watch your form or have a friend join you for support, especially one who is a more regular exerciser than you, as they can inspire you to increase your fitness goals.

7. **Take a morning bike, swim, or outdoor fitness class.**
   Now that the weather is warming up, your local gym or community center may offer outdoor fitness classes such as alfresco spinning and yoga. Seize the opportunity to mix up your environment or try a new activity. Perhaps you'll make some new personal connections and bolster your local support system. Spring is all about newness, which also includes new friends. Swimming and biking are great outdoor activities you can do solo or with a buddy. If you're new to any of these activities, go with a friend, join a group class, or book a lesson so you're sure to set yourself up for success to obtain results and avoid possible injury.

Spring Mindset

Spring is the time for cleansing and initiation, and there are a number of meditations, visualizations, and mindfulness exercises to these ends. Transitioning from winter blues, we can support our hormonal harmony with mindset shifts and practices. We can do breathwork exercises for spring rekindling and to warm the body. This is also the perfect time to start a new creative activity and do some spring-cleaning in our homes.

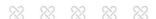

7 Mindset Activities for Spring

1. **Declutter and spring-clean your space.**
   Spring-cleaning can lead to a tidier space and a clearer, calmer mind. A decluttered environment gives us more mental space for clarity and creativity. It also clears out dust laden with toxins that has settled in our homes. Start with one area rather than tackling the entire home and giving up from being overwhelmed. Choose your pantry, desk, a bedroom closet, or a bathroom cabinet as a starting point. When you have one success, it's easier to have more. To get motivated, close your eyes and visualize the end goal of your clean area. Then get going! If you have family or a roommate, get their help and make it a group project to build camaraderie.

2. **Plant seeds.**
   It's never too late to develop a green thumb by starting a garden or nourishing a houseplant. If you have room in your yard, start planting seeds where they'll be protected from deer and other animals and have plenty of sun. Check with a local farmer or search online to find seedlings that grow well in your area, and watch the weather forecast for those spring frosts so you can plan accordingly. If you don't have space or the inclination to start an outdoor garden, tap into the benefits of

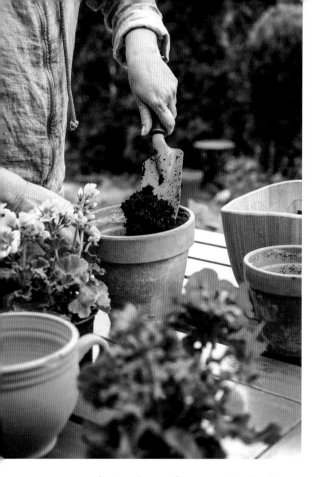

them outdoors. As you move, notice the sights, sounds, and scents of life and rebirth of spring. You may have already checked this off your list with your sunrise hike in the movement section, so find a new location and enjoy again! You may find during your walk that you want to pause and observe your surroundings by simply sitting in nature. Find some trees and enjoy forest bathing (immersing yourself in the forest), which has been shown to help reduce cortisol and blood pressure and improve mood.

4. **Create a candle-lighting ritual.**
   Lighting a candle can represent bringing in the light of spring. Select a candle without synthetic fragrance but rather made from natural ingredients such beeswax, coconut, and soy. Find a peaceful location and think of at least one thing you're grateful for. You may also set an intention for your day or send a blessing for a loved one. With these thoughts in your mind, light your candle. In your journal, write down what you're grateful for, your blessings, and any positive thoughts for springtime that you want to explore.

gardening by tending to a single plant. Anyone who gardens can tell you the joy and sense of accomplishment that comes from watching seeds grow into plants and flourish. If you have children around, encourage their involvement and watch their wonderment in the process. Digging into soil is good for your microbiome, too!

3. **Take a walking meditation in a garden, forest, park, beach, or mountaintop.**
   Many people think meditation has to be done sitting still, but walking meditations can be just as impactful, if not more, especially when you do

5. **Choose one thing to simplify.**
   What can you simplify to revitalize your body, mind, and soul? Consider your daily routine and create a schedule that helps you save time and increase efficiency. You may find there are

things in your life that are drawing more of your energy than they deserve. Are you overcommitted? What can you take off your plate so you have more time to relax? Take a look at your to-do list and remove anything that's unnecessary, drains your energy, or takes up too much of your valuable time. When you let go of something that you no longer need and simplify aspects of your life, you allow space to bring in something new that nourishes your mind and lifts your spirit.

6. **Try something new.**
   Spring is the ideal time to pick up a new hobby, learn to play an instrument, or start a crafty project. Have fun and be creative! Spring is the perfect time to play, and, even better, explore hobbies with a new or rekindled friendship. If you're short on time, start small. Here are some ideas:

   ❀ Create a springtime wreath
   ❀ Grow a windowsill herb garden
   ❀ Have a spa day at home with DIY skincare
   ❀ Make your own fragrance-free natural candles
   ❀ Make a suncatcher
   ❀ Set up a bird feeder and learn about birds in your area
   ❀ Create an outdoor garden mandala, medicine wheel, or other spiritual symbol to help you connect with nature's wisdom

Enjoy these activities alone for nurturing "me" time, or invite your housemates to join in on the fun!

7. **Try a new bedtime relaxation technique.**
   Sleep may be more challenging as the days get sunnier, so start with a relaxation technique to prepare your body and mind for z's. You want to aim for seven to eight hours of sleep every night, so if you have to wake up at 6 AM, you'll want to be in bed and ready for sleep by 10 PM. There are many books, apps, and videos with relaxation techniques to choose from. Here is a simple one to try: While lying in bed, close your eyes and imagine letting go. You can picture a wave gently washing over you and taking away negative thoughts, misunderstandings, judgments, or anything else you wish to release. Take deep breaths, and with each exhale, notice every muscle from head to toe relax as if your body is melting into the mattress beneath you.

Spring Skincare

When spring-cleaning your home, don't forget your vanity and bathroom cabinets. That means tossing out expired personal-care products and making room for new, natural, clean, and organic skincare alternatives. The goal is to make skincare more about self-care than simply applying products to your skin, so embracing the senses brings mindset into your skincare routine. Spring brings more sunshine and typically more humidity, so it's a good time to shift your skincare routine from your winter-time approach, too.

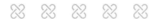

7 Skincare Practices for Spring

1. **Spring-clean your personal-care products.**
    When was the last time you cleaned out your skincare cabinet? Skincare products and makeup do have expiration dates. Spring is the perfect time to bring in the trash bin and toss anything that's over two to three years old. In addition, clean your makeup brushes and facial sponges with some natural soap and warm water. While you're at it, check the ingredient labels of your personal-care products and throw out those that contain any of the twenty toxic ingredients below:

    1. Fragrance
    2. Formaldehyde and formaldehyde releasers (quaternium-15, diazolidinyl urea, DMDM hydantoin, bronopol, or imidazolidinyl urea)
    3. Mineral oil and petroleum (also called petrolatum, petroleum jelly, and paraffin oil)
    4. Parabens (propyl-, isopropyl-, butyl-, and isobutyl-)
    5. Ethanolamines (diethanolamine [DEA], monoethanolamine [MEA], and triethanolamine [TEA])
    6. Oxybenzone (benzophenone), octinoxate, and homosalate
    7. Hydroquinone (or tocopheryl acetate) and other skin lighteners
    8. Butylated hydroxyanisole (BHA)
    9. Triclosan and triclocarban
    10. Coal tar ingredients (including aminophenol, diaminobenzene, and phenylenediamine)
    11. Toluene
    12. Mica, silica (crystalline), talc (unless asbestos-free), and titanium dioxide nanoparticles (TiO2) in powders, loose makeup, or spray
    13. Methylisothiazolinone, methylchloroisothiazolinone, and benzisothiazolinone (also 2-methyl-4-isothiazoline-3-one, Neolone 950, OriStar MIT, and Microcare MT, and 5-Chloro-2-methyl-4-isothiazolin-3-one)
    14. Heavy metals such as mercury, lead, arsenic, and aluminum (calomel, lead acetate, mercurio, mercuric chloride, or thimerosal)
    15. Resorcinol (or 1,3-benzenediol, resorcin, 1,3-dihydroxybenzene, m-hydroxybenzene, m-dihydroxyphenol)
    16. Carbon black (or D&C Black No. 2, channel black, acetylene black, furnace black, lamp black, and thermal black)
    17. P-phenylenediamine (or 4-aminoaniline; 1,4-benzenediamine;

p-diaminobenzene; 1,4-diamino-benzene; 1,4-phenylene diamine)

18. Teflon (and polytetrafluoro-ethylene [PTFE], polyperflu-oromethylisopropyl ether, and DEA-C8-18 perfluoroalkylethyl phosphate)

19. Acrylamide (also polyacrylamide, polyacrylate, polyquaternium, acrylate)

20. Phenoxyethanol (also Euxyl K 400 and PhE)

2. **Ramp up exfoliation to brighten skin.** Your skin should be able to tolerate acids before the summer sun kicks in, but don't overdo it. Nutrient-rich skincare ingredients and formulations can help decrease inflammation and support healthy skin cell turnover, collagen production, and hydration. Vitamin C, for example, can aid in promoting collagen production when used on the skin.[134] Two of my favorite natural ingredients are acerola cherry fruit extract and chlorella (green algae) extract. Acerola cherry fruit extract is a rich source of vitamin C, putting foods commonly known to be high in vitamin C, like oranges and strawberries, to shame. Meanwhile, chlorella extract is a freshwater algae that is known for its potential to purify and energize the skin. Chlorella plays a role in inhibiting the enzymes that break down collagen and elastin.

3. **Use dry skin brushing.** Enhance circulation, help improve detoxification, and exfoliate dead skin with dry skin brushing, which is done prior to bathing. Use a long-handled skin brush, available online or at select health food and specialty stores. If you have irritated skin, open wounds, or severely dry skin, skip this technique or work around affected areas. While your body is dry, start at your toes and brush your skin with your long-handled skin brush in upward strokes toward your heart. Use light to medium pressure, as this should not be painful. When you reach your abdomen, start over at your fingers and brush toward your heart, along your arms and up your back. Continue brushing over your body (except your head and neck) in movements toward your heart. Once you've covered your entire body, enjoy a warm shower and finish with a ten-second cold shower blast and gently pat your skin dry.

4. **Ease off on certain oils and moisturizers.** As the season shifts from cold to warm, move away from using heavy oils and thick moisturizers. Instead, switch to lighter moisturizers with humectants and emollients, and avoid occlusives such as dimethicone, which trap in heat and moisture and may disrupt the skin microbiome. Even as the temperature rises and humidity

increases, your skin can still benefit from moisturizing. Opt for natural and light serums, moisturizers, and plant-based oil blends, such as The Spa Dr.'s steps 2, 3, and 4. Don't skip moisturizing regardless of your skin type.

5. **Update your SPF.**
Now that we're closer to the sun, you need more UV protection than you did in the winter. Consider replacing toxin-laden and pore-clogging foundations with a tinted mineral-based sunscreen. Be sure to check the labels to avoid toxic ingredients such as synthetic fragrance. Take your time adjusting to the sun so you don't burn. Just in case, keep some aloe gel or an aloe plant on hand. If you use retinol products, be sure to use them only at night, and use caution with other photosensitizing ingredients such as citrus and enzymes. Both natural and completely synthetic skincare products can contain ingredients that increase your susceptibility to sun damage. Look for a new cute hat, sun shirts and other cover-ups, and sunglasses to prepare for the sunny days ahead.

6. **Choose skincare products with anti-inflammatory ingredients.**
For many people, springtime means allergies, eczema (atopic dermatitis), and inflamed skin. To help decrease inflammation and reduce sensitivity

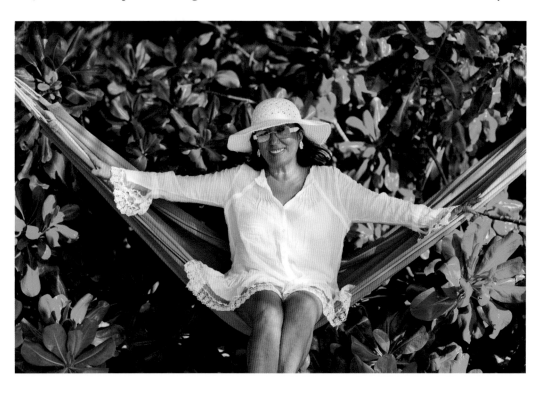

and irritation, choose natural skincare products with soothing ingredients. For example, sunflower oil is soothing and hydrating, even for sensitive skin. Green, white, and rooibos teas also provide calm and moisturize skin while providing antioxidants. Adaptogenic herbs like ginseng root extract can be used topically to de-stress skin.

7. **Go light on the makeup.**
   As the temperature and humidity rise, your pores are more likely to clog, and the combination of heat and makeup can disrupt your skin's microbiota. Once you've cleaned out your personal-care bags and cabinets, look for more natural, spring-focused, and light alternatives. Ideally, your skin will be so healthy and vibrant that you'll have nothing to hide, and makeup is only something you reach for to enhance your natural beauty on special occasions. If you're still working on clearing up and balancing your skin's glow, try to ease your way off the heavy foundations and concealers so your skin can adjust and heal while you're addressing root causes from the inside and out.

CHAPTER 11

SUMMER RESET

(June, July, and August)

Live in the sunshine, swim the sea, drink the wild air.

—Ralph Waldo Emerson

Summer is the season of sun, longer days, and shorter nights. Nature is in full swing—from bees buzzing and birds chirping to thunderstorms booming and rainbows painting the sky in watercolor hues. Many types of flowers are in full bloom, and summer fruit is deliciously ripe and abundant. With longer days that are warm, we're spending more time outdoors and taking vacations, so our mood and vitality is typically much more elevated than during other times of year. We don't have to worry about bundling up in clothing and protective gear to shield ourselves from cold weather; instead, our wardrobe is easy-breezy.

Due to more sunlight exposure, summer is the time when conditions are optimal for plants' photosynthesis, and, in exchange, plants are giving us more oxygen to help us breathe and live. All of this allows us to embrace the exuberance the summer setting provides, and derive nutrients from food and sunlight. It's the time to tap into the energy that abounds so we can restore our bodies and be prepared for the coming winter.

Ideally, this season's seven-day reset will start on or around the summer solstice (usually June 20 or 21), the longest day of the year. It's when the sun is shining on us the longest, which creates the perfect time for getting outdoors and being active.

Important shifts occur with our hormones in summer that account for changes in our mood and behaviors. For women looking to get pregnant, summer is the ultimate time of year for conception because research shows a trend toward higher levels of follicle-stimulating hormone and greater frequency of ovulation compared to wintertime.[135] Menstruating women may notice that their cycle is slightly shorter in summer. Postmenopausal women have peak levels of total and free estradiol (the active form of estrogen) in June, which may provide an opportunity for a boost in estrogen's benefits.[136]

Because estrogen has a facilitatory role on dopamine, it may help give you a positive sense of pleasure in the sunnier months. More sunshine also means a boost in our serotonin levels, which means we're more likely to have a brighter outlook in summer months.[137]

Summer is also a time to soak up the sun and get your vitamin D fix. While we've become wary of too much sun exposure for good reason (no one wants skin cancer or a surplus of wrinkles), there is a healthy balance for flourishing in the sun. Natural sunlight is our main source of vitamin D, and wearing sunscreen of SPF 30 reduces the body's ability to make vitamin D by more than 95 percent.[138]

Summer Food

Because of the abundance of plants growing under the full sun, the focus of food during the summer reset is mostly sun-loving, nutrient-rich produce. Late spring through summer is the best time for cheese production,

as well. Grass-fed cows, goats, and sheep are grazing on rich grass, clover, herbs, and flowers, so the nutritional content and flavor of their milk is at its peak. Fresh trout are most prolific in spring and summer, and it's best to eat wild salmon in late spring through summer because it's when they've completed their life cycle, making it a more sustainable time to catch them.

With warmer temperatures, we also want more cooling foods like cucumber, watermelon, cantaloupe, cilantro, and parsley. Avoid foods like winter squash and warming foods like hot peppers, ginger, and cinnamon during hot days. Swap out hot drinks for cool water and iced herbal teas to keep your body's internal temperature balanced.

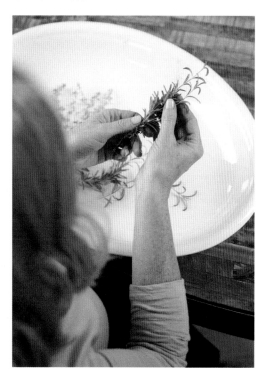

If you tend toward conditions that reflect rising internal heat such as rosacea and hot flashes, you'll want to avoid spicy foods like jalapeños and cayenne, which can worsen your symptoms. Women with these conditions already have a predisposition to being triggered by these foods, and the heat of summer months can make it worse. During perimenopause, temperature regulation can be more challenging, so be mindful of supporting your body by eating cooling foods and herbs this time of year.

For additional seasonal foods, check with your local farmers market to find out which produce is freshest where you live. Choose organic and nongenetically modified foods as much as possible.

Foods most abundant during summer include:

❊   Grains: Since summer is a time of plentiful fruit and vegetables, it's the perfect time to shift away from grains, with the exception of an occasional nongenetically modified corn on the cobb.

CORN (NON-GMO)

❊   Fruits: While some health experts recommend a low-fruit diet, summer is the ideal time to enjoy fruit since it is rich in flavor and nourishment, and the summer heat and outdoor activities increase our need for nutrients naturally found in fresh fruit.

AVOCADOS	FIGS	PEACHES
BLACKBERRIES	GRAPES	PINEAPPLE
BLUEBERRIES	HONEYDEW MELON	PLUMS
BOYSENBERRIES	MULBERRIES	RASPBERRIES
CANTALOUPE	NECTARINES	STRAWBERRIES
CHERRIES	PASSION FRUIT	WATERMELON
(early summer)		

❉ Vegetables: When the temperatures rise, it may be harder to find certain vegetables, so we focus on heat-resistant crops and those that grow above ground.

ARUGULA	HEAT-RESISTANT SUMMER GREENS	SUMMER SQUASH (zucchini, yellow squash)
CUCUMBER	(malabar spinach, lamb's-quarters, chicory leaves, and sorrel)	TOMATILLOS
EGGPLANT		TOMATOES
OKRA	RHUBARB	
PURSLANE		

❉ Legumes: Summer is the perfect time to enjoy fresh seasonal legumes as a protein and fiber source.

BLACK-EYED PEAS	GARBANZO BEANS	LIMA BEANS
FAVA BEANS	GREEN BEANS	

❉ Nuts and seeds: Coconuts grow in the tropics and subtropics and most abundantly in the warmest months. However, it's rarely grown where many of us in the US live. If you're lucky to live in a place where it grows, that's great! With so many other foods in season in summer, you can eat fewer nuts and seeds and focus on other sources of proteins and fats.

COCONUTS	MACADAMIA NUTS	PEANUTS

TIP: Find ways to maximize your time and minimize prep. For example, make more than a recipe calls for and set aside as leftovers or chop a few days' worth of vegetables and fruit and store in a glass or ceramic container in the refrigerator.

❖ Animal protein: Summer is the time to enjoy dairy, particularly goat and sheep cheese because it's when the flavor and availability is highest. It is also an excellent time to find wild Alaskan salmon and freshwater trout.

FRESHWATER TROUT	LAMB	WILD ALASKAN
GOAT AND SHEEP	(late summer)	SALMON
CHEESE		

❖ Herbs and spices: Spice up your summer meals with cooling and flavorful fresh seasonal herbs.

BASIL	ROSEMARY
CILANTRO	SAGE
MINT	SHALLOTS
PARSLEY	

❖ Sweets: Stevia plants grow easiest in summer, so you can enjoy a leaf in your smoothie. Later in summer, seek out a local beekeeper for fresh honey.

HONEY	STEVIA
(late summer)	(early summer)

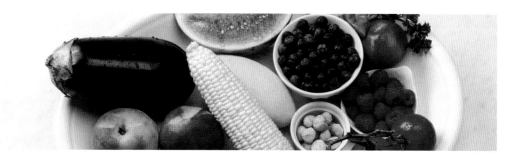

SAMPLE SUMMER
MEAL IDEAS FROM RECIPES

Here are a week's worth of ideas to help you get started on the 7-Day Natural Beauty Reset for summer. Feel free to modify, substitute, and repeat recipes throughout. Remember, this is not about restriction or limitations; it's about enjoying the flavors and nourishment available during the season you're in. Make note of which meals you enjoy the most so you can continue making them throughout the summer season.

SAMPLE DAY 1

BREAKFAST: Peach Coconut Mint Smoothie (page 209)

LUNCH: Cucumber Salad (page 217)

DINNER: Wild Alaskan Salmon with Pesto Green Beans (page 212)

SNACKS/SWEETS: Roasted Tomatillo Salsa (page 224) and GMO-free corn chips

SAMPLE DAY 2

BREAKFAST: Green Goddess Smoothie (page 211)

LUNCH: Salmon Salad (find the recipe with the Salmon Cabbage Salad recipe on page 186) from leftover salmon and serve over summer greens

DINNER: Lamb Chops with Mint Chutney (page 215)

SNACKS/SWEETS: Coconut Ice Cream (page 221)

SAMPLE DAY 3

BREAKFAST: Berry Bliss Smoothie Bowl (page 210)

LUNCH: Watermelon Salad with Mint and Goat Feta (page 213)

DINNER: Macadamia-Crusted Trout with Pineapple Chutney (page 216)

SNACKS/SWEETS: Creamy Chocolate Mousse Parfait (page 222)

SAMPLE DAY 4

BREAKFAST: Golden Mango Smoothie (page 211)

LUNCH: Tomato and Peach Summer Salad (page 218)

DINNER: Ratatouille (page 220)

SNACKS/SWEETS: Summer Berry Crisp (page 223)

SAMPLE DAY 5

BREAKFAST: Make your own smoothie bowl with one serving of seasonal fruit, one serving of summer veggies, one serving of nuts, and 1 cup of water or unsweetened coconut nut milk

LUNCH: Leftover Ratatouille

DINNER: Make your own grilled zucchini, eggplant, and shiitake mushrooms topped with goat feta and lamb meatballs made from ground lamb

SNACKS/SWEETS: Make your own frozen seasonal berries on a skewer

SAMPLE DAY 6

BREAKFAST: Make your own smoothie with one seasonal fruit, 1 cup of summer veggies, one serving of nuts, and 1 cup of water or unsweetened coconut nut milk

LUNCH: Summer Gazpacho (page 217)

DINNER: Summer Squash Tacos (page 219)

SNACKS/SWEETS: Melon with Coconut Sauce (page 224)

SAMPLE DAY 7

BREAKFAST: Make your own smoothie with one serving of seasonal fruit, one serving of summer veggies, one serving of nuts, and 1 cup of water or unsweetened coconut milk

LUNCH: Summer Greens Salad with Black-Eyed Peas (page 214)

DINNER: Leftover Summer Gazpacho

SNACKS/SWEETS: Make your own variation of Nut Crackers with Black Bean Dip (page 188) by adding Basil Pesto (find the recipe in the Wild Alaskan Salmon with Pesto Green Beans recipe on page 212)

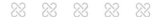

ADDITIONAL SNACK IDEAS FOR SUMMER

- Fruit salad (any combination of blackberries, blueberries, raspberries, strawberries, mulberries, boysenberries, grapes, nectarines, peaches, cantaloupe, honeydew melon, cherries [early summer], figs, pineapple, plums, passion fruit, or watermelon); for extra flavor, sprinkle with stevia powder and shredded coconut
- Herbal iced tea with fresh mint and stevia leaves
- Macadamia nuts
- Fresh coconut (cut open the top, drink the water, and scoop out the meat)
- Frozen fruit pops (blend any combination of the summer fruits and then pour into an ice tray with toothpicks or into popsicle molds and freeze)
- Nut crackers with smoked salmon

Summer Movement

Because this is the most active time of the year and the days are the longest, we want to enjoy the great outdoors with more gusto. Therefore, it's the perfect time for increasing physical activity. Regardless of your current fitness level, now is the time to use the great outdoors for motivation. Enjoy nature and spend time doing new or familiar activities such as hiking, biking, swimming, surfing, and trail running. Because summer days can quickly heat up, do your best to exercise in the morning or evenings.

Don't forget to grab your water before you head out. Remember that water is often a common source of contaminants such as lead, arsenic, pesticides, and even medications, so you want to always choose filtered. Add liquid or powdered electrolytes when exercising outdoors and when temperatures are high.

If you're exercising outdoors, don't forget your sun protection and remember to reapply more frequently as perspiration and water activities can cause your sunscreen to rub off more easily. Remember that mineral-based sunscreens provide a great barrier protection, but once they wear off, they're no longer helping you. If you use a spray, ensure it's free of oxybenzone and nanosized particles and be sure to rub it into your skin after applying so it's evenly distributed and covering your skin.

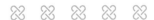

7 Movements for Summer

1. **Do cooling yoga poses.**
    Yoga offers benefits for every season, and in the summer we can focus on shifting into postures that cool and calm our bodies. We're less likely to experience stiffness in the summer, so it can be a great time to start yoga or push your poses a bit further. Still, be mindful not to overdo it because that's when injuries happen. Yoga outdoors can be a nice alternative, and, again, opt for a morning or evening class so you're not doing your practice in the sweltering heat. Otherwise, opt for a well-ventilated indoor class to avoid overheating.

    Here are some cooling and calming yoga poses to look for online or in a yoga class:

    - Moon salutations (a variation of sun salutations)
    - Cat-cow pose
    - Supine spinal twist pose
    - Legs up the wall
    - Downward-facing dog

2. **Try an outdoor bootcamp.**
    While the weather is sunny, it's the perfect time to create your own bootcamp in your driveway or backyard. You can use trees, shrubs, or two cones to indicate your destination spots for sprints and lunges and create a course. Here's an example you can repeat several times for an outdoor bootcamp:

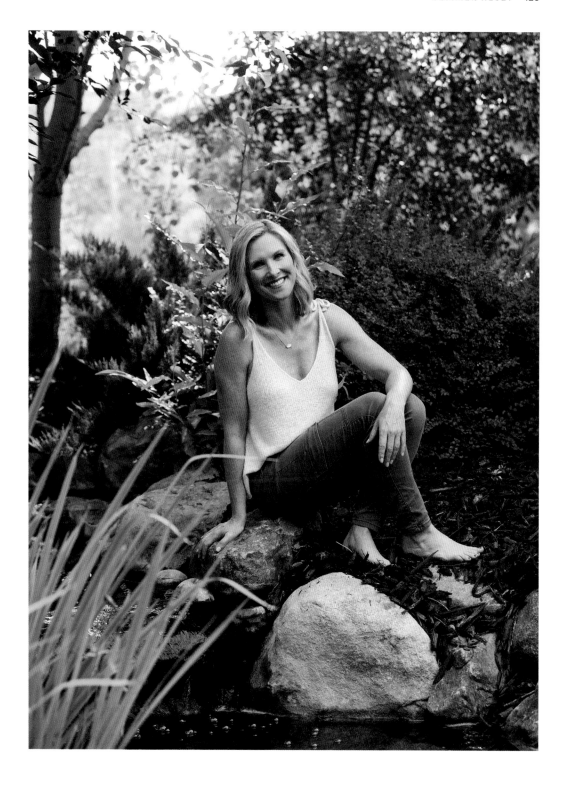

- 5–10 Side Steps in each direction
- Jump Rope or High Knees March for 10–30 seconds
- 20 Throw Punches (alternately punch the air like there's a punching bag in front of you)
- 5–10 Lunges in each direction

3. **Seek an outdoor sport.**
Set your alarm and get to a court or field early. Bring friends or join others for activities such as volleyball, tennis, pickleball, badminton, golf, flag football, ultimate Frisbee, or softball. This is a great opportunity for community building because in summer months you may feel more outgoing and lively. Some days you may still feel like doing a solo sweat session. Don't let that stop you—go for a bike ride or a swim. Whoever you're with and whichever sport you choose, set yourself up for success and bring the appropriate gear, wearing a hat and moisture-wicking clothing to help keep your temperature balanced. Also, keep applying your sunscreen and stay hydrated with filtered electrolyte water.

4. **Create a playground or park workout.**
Mix up your workout environment and bring out your inner kid by taking your movement to a local park or playground. If you have children, bring them along for the fun. Get creative! For example, try booty-toning squats using a playground bench, or do a little high-intensity interval training by sprinting up and down playground stairs. In a park, soak up the benefits of being in nature while getting your heart rate up. You may find there's no shortage of inspiration. A word of caution: be mindful of your form and fitness level, and don't push yourself too hard. A new setting may mean a higher risk for injury.

Here's an example of a playground workout. Choose three to five exercises and repeat two to five times:

- Two to five minutes walking or running up and down stairs
- Ten to twenty triceps dips using a park bench
- Ten to twenty squats or lunges using a park bench
- Ten to twenty swing body weight rows (hold a swing in front of you, step forward so your body is at an angle tilting back, and then with your arms pull your upper body toward the swing)
- Ten to twenty swing squat hops (hold the swing in front of you, step back until there's tension, squat, and then jump)
- Bonus: Try some chin-ups on the monkey bars—even if it's just one!

5. **Plan a social fitness hour.**
Bond with your support system by combining a gathering like a barbecue or cookout with fitness. Do this by

suggesting a pre- or post-party walk, hike, or outdoor group fitness class such as yoga. Choose a location near a park, forest, beach, or backyard, so you can easily shift from party mode to your fitness activity, or vice versa. If you're planning to indulge in food and alcohol, exercise before your get-together—this will ensure you fit it in. If you and your guests plan to eat and drink in moderation, exercise after the get-together—doing so will help improve digestion, burn calories, and balance blood sugar for a more stable mood. Regardless of your workout timing, keep the entire event healthy (and your guests well-nourished) by whipping up a seasonal summer salad or grilled food from the recipes section.

6. **Hit the water.**
Cool off under the sun by taking your workout to the water such as a lake, river, or ocean. Then pick an activity that strikes your fancy. Options include swimming, stand-up paddle boarding, body surfing or full-out surfing, water aerobics, wakeboarding, wakesurfing, waterskiing, kneeboarding, kiteboarding, canoeing, kayaking, or sailing. You can rent, borrow, or bring your own gear.

While you're cooling off in the water, you'll be getting in exercise and boosting feel-good neurotransmitters. In one study with eighty sixty-five-year-olds, participants noticed physical health benefits after doing ten weeks of aquatic exercise compared to the same amount of land-based workouts. And a review of eighteen studies showed that water-based exercise improves mood, depression, anxiety, and balance.[139] If you're new to the activity, be prepared to rent equipment and strongly consider using a trained instructor for guidance. As always with outdoor exercise, grab your sunscreen and plenty of water.

7. **Stretch in the shade of a tree.**
You may be feeling more energetic in summer compared to other seasons, but don't forget to take time to rest and restore as well as stretch before and after your workout. To reap the benefits of the outdoors, do these practices with a tree as your prop, for either shade or a structure to deepen your stretch.

Here is some inspiration:

* Legs up the tree
* Side bends with one hand on the tree and the other stretching up and toward the tree (and then alternate sides)
* Calf stretches (face the tree with arms straight and palms flat against tree, walk your feet back until you can find an angle of your body where feet are flat and you feel a gentle stretch in your calves)

* Forward fold by keeping your feet hip-distance apart, and lowering the top half of your body forward, trying to touch your lower legs, your toes, or the ground with your fingertips

Summer Mindset

Summer is typically a time of travel and outdoor fun, but take time to be mindful when you can. Remember that mindset isn't just a solo practice, though. Especially in the summertime, take the opportunity to connect with your community while you self-reflect.

Mindfulness practices can bring about a sense of calm and are easy to incorporate into your day while other practices may make you feel a bit out of your comfort zone. Trying something new that may be challenging is important for growth and well-being. While your mood is elevated, let go of your inhibitions and step out of your comfort zone!

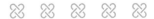

7 Mindset Activities for Summer

1. **Retreat to the trees for forest bathing.**
   Bring a blanket or a camping chair and find some shade under the trees to relax and enjoy the healing powers of trees. You may want to bring some natural bug repellent, such as one containing citronella essential oil.

   If you live in a city, find a few trees to linger under. If you have a car, make the drive to a forest for deeper immersion. Try a walking meditation, turn off your ruminations, and take in your surroundings—smell the earth, leaf, and pine cone scents as they waft around you. Look for signs of wildlife and notice the colors of the plants. Listen to the breeze through the trees and any birds that may be chirping. Take this time for healing by reconnecting with yourself and nature.

2. **Enjoy longer meditations (twenty minutes or more).**
   Find a quiet location in your home or outdoors without distractions. Set your alarm if you have limited time so you don't have to wonder what time it is, which can take you out of your meditative state. Focus on something—a mantra, a candle flame, a song, or your breath—and allow your to-do list, concerns, worries, and stressors to slip away. To settle into your meditation, take some deep, cleansing breaths and feel your body relax and negative thoughts wash away.

3. **Reframe your body awareness.**
   With warmer temperatures of summer, we're wearing less clothing and exposing more skin. We may notice body image issues coming to the surface. If this describes you, know this is a very human experience that we all have. When you catch yourself being critical of your skin or body parts after putting

on your bathing suit, shorts, or sundress, take a moment to acknowledge your thoughts. Instead of immediately suppressing your feelings or spiraling into negative self-talk, pause and observe without judgment. Remember, you're not alone—this is a common human experience. Then try to reframe your perspective. Instead of being pained by the physical attributes you dislike, attempt to see them as traits that make you unique. Identify and focus on the parts of your body you do like. Find some positive messages for yourself and write them down in your journal. For example, you could write, "I am enough, I am beautiful the way I am, my body is capable of amazing and powerful things." I hope you feel comfortable writing these down because they're 100 percent true for all of us.

4. **Garden.**
   Whether it's your own garden or a friend's or community's garden, spend time today with your hands in the soil, touching plants under the warm sun. You can get a nice dose of vitamin D while you're fueling your creativity and reconnecting with nature.

   Research shows that gardening helps with cognition, mood, sleep, stress management, and healthy weight maintenance. This can be as active or as meditative as you'd like. For a bit of a workout, exert yourself with some digging, shoveling, raking, or hauling. Or for more relaxing downtime, find a place to kneel or sit and pot, weed, trim, pick plants, or plant seeds. To support a sense of connection, join others in a family, community, or school organic garden. Use natural alternatives to pesticides and herbicides to reduce your exposure to EDCs and other toxic chemicals. Wear gloves, closed-toe shoes, long pants, and other clothing to protect your skin.

5. **Breathe to cool and calm.**
   On hot summer days, we can use certain breathing techniques to cool and calm ourselves. If you feel hot and overstimulated, find a relaxing position such as legs up the wall. Be aware of your breathing and then slow it down to a five-count inhale followed by a five-count exhale. For more of a cooling breath, try single-nostril breathing by plugging your right nostril and breathing in and out only through the left nostril. If you're seeking more balance, try alternating your breath through each nostril by closing one nostril at a time and breathing through the other side, as described in the fall activities section. To quickly dispel heat, try lion's breath, where you inhale and tighten the muscles in your face and then exhale while sticking out your tongue, opening your eyes wide, and rolling them upward. Repeat this three or more times.

6. **Create a community project to give back.**
Summer is an excellent time for building community while friends and neighbors are spending more time outdoors in their yards, having barbecues and block parties, picnicking in the park, playing with kids at the playground, and walking their dogs around the block. Now is the time to connect with others to find a way to give back.

If you aren't sure where to start, think of what your community may need and ask your neighbors for their input. Then start a community project to give back for that cause. Here are some ideas:

- Initiate a street cleanup
- Create a green or open space
- Start a community garden
- Collect clothing and supplies for those in need
- Organize errand-running for elders
- Ramp up the local recycling program
- Create a healthy cooking, baking, or arts-and-crafts group that gives back
- Join a book club with a charitable component
- Participate in your local church or spiritual group's projects of giving
- Participate in an organized bike ride, run, hike, or walk for a cause

Any of these opportunities offer a great way to make friends, expand your social support, and contribute to your community!

7. **Take a trip to explore nature you haven't seen.**
We tend to be creatures of habit and walk the same trails, go to the same parks, and wade in the same waters time and again. But trying new things and seeing new sights helps boost memory, concentration, and focus as we age. Getting outdoors and breathing fresh air also boosts our mood and gives our bodies a break from the toxins we're exposed to indoors. Find a place in nature you haven't explored and plan a date to go. It could be a secret neighborhood spot that you discover or it could be a new hiking trail, beach, or lake. You can do a search online or take it a step further and ask neighbors and friends for ideas because these hidden gems aren't always listed in a travel book or on a website. You may even want to plan an extended weekend getaway or a camping trip for a nature excursion that is new for you and your partner, the whole family, or a group of friends. Our planet is full of natural wonders to explore!

Summer Skincare

With sun exposure at its highest, it's essential to achieve the right balance of sun protection with sunscreen and cover-ups. Too much sun exposure can lead to damaging effects and accelerate premature skin aging. Summer is a great time for your yearly dermatologist appointment to check for any precancerous or cancerous skin lesions.

You also want to keep your skin hydrated and soothe irritated skin. If you spend time in a pool, the exposure to chlorine or salt can cause drying and temporary irritation. Spending too much time in air conditioning also dries out skin. On the other hand, being outdoors with heat causes more sweating, which can lead to clogged pores and breakouts. The key is balance so your skin feels hydrated and soothed without feeling oily and sticky.

Summer is also a common time for itchy rashes from plants, bug bites, cuts, bruises, and scrapes from all your summer fun. Reaching for natural ingredients that help heal and soothe will ensure your skin stays happy through the season.

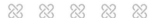

7 Skincare Practices for Summer

1. **Use a face mist.**
   DIY face mists and premade formulations with natural ingredients can provide a refreshing and hydrating boost to your skin's summer needs. Rose water, cucumber, and mint are some of my favorite cooling and soothing ingredients for summer face mists. (See Cucumber Mint Face Mist recipe.) For another refreshing option, you can make herbal and green tea face mists, and chill them. Be sure to use distilled water and refrigerate between uses to help reduce the growth of bacteria in DIY recipes.

If you choose a face mist that's already made, check the label to ensure it doesn't contain potentially harmful ingredients such as synthetic fragrance. Remember that organic essential oils are an excellent alternative. Anything that you spray in the air can make its way into your lungs, so it's not just your skin you're watching out for. As always, it's best to do a skin patch test, especially if you have sensitive skin.

2. **Wear a hat and other sun cover-ups in addition to an SPF of at least 30.**
   Don't forget your lips, ears, and the exposed areas of your scalp and other parts of your body.

   The sun's damaging rays are at their peak in the summer months, so do everything you can to protect yourself while enjoying the beautiful outdoors. Don't hide away indoors. There are many options for sun hats, clothing, and mineral-based sunscreens that will do the trick. You don't have to cover every spot of your skin all summer long. You can enjoy soaking up vitamin D to build up your stores. Take some time to expose your skin to sunlight in the early and later parts of the day without wearing sunscreen on your arms, legs, and other areas where you get less sun exposure. Because your face, neck, and the tops of your hands get the year-round UV rays, those are the areas to keep protected as much as possible in the summer sun.

3. **Start a natural skincare routine and create a first-aid kit.**

   Bites, stings, scratches, scrapes, bumps, and burns are part of summer, especially if you have children and are enjoying an active outdoorsy lifestyle. Be prepared for potential mishaps. A basic first aid kit is always a good idea to have in your home, car, and recreational vehicles, and you can step up your kit with some natural additions. Here are some of my favorites to keep on hand for summer's acute skin issues:

   * Aloe vera gel—great for minor burns (make sure it's 100 percent natural)
   * Calendula spray—for minor cuts and scrapes (make sure you choose a non-alcoholic version so it doesn't burn)
   * Arnica gel or cream—for bumps and bruises
   * Healing salve with comfrey, plantain, and vitamin E—for cuts and scrapes
   * Baking soda—for insect bites and stings; make a paste with baking soda and water to stop the sting
   * Epsom salt—to soothe sore muscles in a soak
   * Lavender essential oil—a few drops in a spray bottle with distilled water can help sooth minor burns and skin irritations

4. **Avoid heat-trapping ingredients in personal-care products.**

   When the temperatures are high, allow your body to perspire and be free of heat-trapping ingredients like dimethicone and other occlusives, which are known to create a barrier on the surface of skin to trap in moisture. While these ingredients can give your skin a dewy, moisturized look, they tend to trap heat, which may lead to irritation and breakouts. Your skin doesn't breathe in the way your lungs exchange oxygen, but it does need exposure to air and light, and an ability to easily perspire. Look for these ingredients in your makeup, lotion, and sunscreen. And then turn your attention to your underarms. Antiperspirants are not a healthy option because they block perspiration (one of the main ways we detox and cool off), and research has shown that they can actually produce more of the malodorous-producing bacteria.[140] Instead, look for natural deodorant alternatives.

DIY Deodorant

INGREDIENTS:

- ½ cup coconut oil
- ½ cup shea or cocoa butter
- 3 to 4 tablespoons baking soda
- ½ cup organic arrowroot powder
- 10 to 20 drops essential oils, such as lavender, frankincense, or rose

Blend all together and place in a mold. Use as needed.

5. **Use a facial sponge with your cleanser.**
    Summer skin can feel sticky and
    harder to cleanse. It's important to
    clean your skin, but be sure to do it
    in a way that protects and nourishes
    rather than strips away naturally occur-
    ring beneficial oils. Resist the tempta-
    tion to switch to foamy cleansers with
    a high pH that damage your skin's
    natural barrier function. Staying away
    from high-pH cleansers will help you
    avoid skin irritation, breakouts, and
    damage from sun and air pollutants.
    Instead, keep using your fabulous oil-
    based cleanser, but use it with warm
    water and a gentle facial sponge or
    washcloth. My favorite is the konjac
    facial sponge, like the one we sell at
    TheSpaDr.com, because when it's wet,
    it's the perfect soft yet exfoliating tex-
    ture to remove your cleanser, makeup,
    perspiration, and other buildup from
    the summer days and nights. Plus,
    konjac is a natural fiber that is biode-
    gradable and compostable. Be sure to
    check the ingredients to make sure it's
    100 percent natural and has no other
    added ingredients, and clean it once a
    week by dropping it into boiled water
    for a minute or two.

6. **Soothe skin with light moisturizers.**
    Well-designed moisturizers protect
    your skin from irritation, dryness, and
    pollution. Even on hot, steamy nights,
    don't skip your moisturizer—but seek
    out a light formulation with plant-
    based ingredients. Specifically, antioxi-
    dants can help protect against the free
    radical damage, and adaptogens help
    de-stress your skin. And check that the
    formulas are in the ideal pH zone to
    help keep your skin glowing today and
    for years to come.

7. **Exfoliate regularly but avoid photo-
    sensitizing ingredients.**
    Exfoliation is important all year long,
    and summer is no exception. The trick
    is that you want to use only photo-
    sensitizing ingredients such as retinol
    and AHAs at night, and avoid the
    more abrasive exfoliants that can make
    your skin feel raw and exposed. You
    can use a gently exfoliating cleanser
    to remove mineral sunscreens, dirt,
    perspiration, and makeup. Or you can
    blend a natural exfoliant with a natural
    cleanser to get the same effect in one
    step. In summer months, I love com-
    bining The Spa Dr.'s Pearl and Rose
    Petal Exfoliant with the Step 1 Gentle
    Cleaners because it gives my skin that
    smooth, hydrated, and deep cleanse it
    craves. You can also try one of the DIY
    cleanser and exfoliant combinations
    you'll find in the recipe section.

CHAPTER 12

PERSONALIZING THE 7-DAY NATURAL BEAUTY RESET

The results of the 7-Day Natural Beauty Reset will start with the first season and rekindle every time you do the next seasonal seven-day reset. You'll be more inclined to follow healthy habits because balanced hormones help your mood, metabolism, and motivation, which also shows up on your skin.

After each season's seven-day reset, take note of your skin and your outer reflection of overall health. You may have already experienced people commenting on your vibrant, healthy glow. But what do you notice? Do you have less darkness and puffiness under your eyes, diminished fine lines, more even skin tone, more vibrant color, or more hydrated or smoother skin? Positive outcomes in these areas are what many of my patients have noticed, and my goal is for you to experience similar results.

After you've studied your skin, step back and notice how you *feel*—because that's where true natural beauty resides. If you're like my patients, you'll notice the healthy glow on your skin *and* a difference in your mood and hormonal well-being.

134

Take my thirty-nine-year-old patient Becky, who after following my program beamed about her healthy skin and was relieved she could consistently get a solid night's sleep and have pain-free regular cycles. Without the fatigue and time she had to take off work due to menstrual pain, she had more energy and enthusiasm to restore her relationship with her husband and get a new job she loved. She was radiating confidence!

This kind of natural beauty and confidence is what I expect for you, too. In this chapter, I will guide you through personalizing the 7-Day Natural Beauty Reset to meet your unique needs. I have included a series of questions divided into categories to help determine which modifications and supplements to consider adding into your routine. The goal is to bring the aforementioned insights and practices all together, helping you achieve and enjoy a lifetime of natural beauty and radiance.

Lifestyle and Environment

Do you live in the northern or southern hemisphere?

If you live in the northern hemisphere, the best time to do the spring 7-Day Natural Beauty Reset is March, and the best time for the fall 7-Day Natural Beauty Reset is September.

If you live in the southern hemisphere, it's the opposite—the best time to do the spring 7-Day Natural Beauty Reset is September, and the best time for the fall 7-Day Natural Beauty Reset is March.

Are there no distinct seasons where you live?

Regardless, following the 7-Day Natural Beauty Reset program can help your body restore balance. It's nice to change your routine, and seasonal transitions are the perfect times to do it. Following a seasonal plan helps us shift and achieve a new process every few months, even if your climate remains the same. I recommend following the seasons for the hemisphere where you reside.

Are you a vegetarian?

If you don't eat meat, you can still follow the 7-Day Natural Beauty Reset because the majority of the recipes and recommendations are (or can be modified to become) plant based. Most of our nutrition comes from plants, but there are certain nutrients, such as iron, zinc, vitamin B_{12}, and omega-3 fatty acids, that are easiest to obtain from animal sources. Therefore, I recommend eating clean sources of animal protein when possible. If it's not, or you have a philosophical reason or aversion to eating meat, consider supplementing with a multivitamin and mineral supplement, or take individual nutrients containing iron (if and while you're still menstruating) and vitamin B_{12}. Source your protein from nuts, seeds, and legumes, especially if you are vegan—that is, if you're avoiding all animal products, including dairy and eggs. If you do eat dairy and eggs, you'll receive some vitamin B_{12} and protein from them. These nutrients are crucial for hormonal balance.

Do you live in an urban environment?

Many of us live in cities, where nature isn't easily accessible. Nature is visually beautiful, and when we include our other senses, such as hearing, smelling, tasting, and feeling, we can experience health benefits.[141] Studies show that being in contact with nature is associated with reduced stress, better sleep, lessened depression and anxiety, enhanced feelings of happiness and satisfaction with life, eased aggression, reduced ADHD symptoms, lower blood

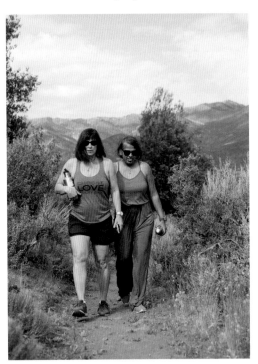

pressure, improved recovery from surgery, reduced pain, enhanced immune function, and a reduced risk for obesity and diabetes (to name a few benefits!).[142]

Because you have less nature around you, you'll want to make some extra effort to reconnect with the outdoors on a daily, monthly, and seasonal basis. Simple adjustments, such as taking walks to a nearby park, rethinking your window coverings to allow more natural light, creating window herb gardens, and finding local sources of plant-based foods to boost your nutrition, can help you restore harmony in your urban dwelling.

Do your work, hobbies, or learning environment cause you to be in front of a computer screen or other electronic device most of the day?

If so, it's time for a nature boost to prevent any potentially damaging effects of overuse of electronics. Take time throughout the day to step away from your computer, phone, or other energy-zapping device and step into nature. Even if it's just a quick walk around the block or park, a few moments in the sun and fresh air can boost your vitamin D and mood, not to mention promote mindfulness. Most of us need this reset, but it's important to realize when you're particularly susceptible to imbalances in your chemical messengers, and make the shifts in your seven-day reset to help restore your harmony with natural rhythms.

Do you consume sugar, fast food, alcohol, caffeine, tobacco, or recreational drugs regularly?

If you consume any of the above substances on a regular basis, this program is a great opportunity to pause ingesting these items for each seasonal reset. Even if it's just to cut them back or out for a week, you'll obtain more benefits from the program without them. Write in your journal how these eliminations affect your mental and physical health. Many of my patients have noticed a reduction in symptoms such as hot flashes, night sweats, and painful periods. Your body's liver and neurological system have to work overtime to process these substances, impairing your body's ability to metabolize hormones and balance your chemical messengers. Taking a break from these habits allows your body to heal.

Skin

Do you have atopic dermatitis (eczema), rosacea, seborrheic dermatitis, acne, or another chronic inflammatory skin condition?

If so, the seasonal recommendations in this book will help because they curb inflammation and optimize skin and gut microbiomes, which play a role in symptoms of these conditions. Making food and skincare modifications can help restore skin to its healthy state. Research has also shown that supplements with a combination of active flavonoids and proteoglycans can be helpful for managing inflammatory conditions.[143] In addition to following this program, there are supplements, such as curcumin, omega-3 fatty acids, zinc, vitamin C, and quercetin, to help give you an antioxidant boost and decrease inflammation. You can find additional recommendations in my book *Clean Skin from Within*.

Are you in the sun every day, or do you have a history of sunburns or going to tanning beds?

First, if you're still lying in the sun to tan or in tanning beds, I encourage you to stop. No longer are we in the days of putting baby oil on your skin to tan (goodbye, 1980s!), which we now know led to significant sun damage, increasing the risk for skin cancers and accelerated skin aging. Don't avoid the sun; instead, find balance. That is, enjoy your dose of vitamin D, yet wear hats and protective clothing and a zinc oxide–based sunscreen. If you do happen to get too much sun, soothe your skin with aloe- and other plant-based oils to nourish and replenish your skin. Consider taking an antioxidant supplement such as astaxanthin or resveratrol to protect your skin from the inside out and possibly help reverse any oxidative damage from excess exposure to damaging UV rays. Melatonin also appears to have a protective role against ultraviolet radiation and mitochondrial dysfunction, so be sure to get a good night's sleep and consider supplementing.[144]

Is your skin showing accelerated signs of aging (age spots, wrinkles, and sagging skin)?

Fine lines and wrinkles are signs that we've been living and laughing, but when we have them prematurely or in excess, it can be a sign that our collagen is breaking down too rapidly. Part of the reason these signs pop up may be related to genetics, but much of it has to do with lifestyle. Follow the seasonal skincare adjustments to protect your skin's collagen, support a healthy mindset, and make time for movement to de-stress as well as consume foods and supplements to boost your nutrition and help slow signs of aging. Consider nourishing your skin externally with The Spa Dr. skincare and consuming antioxidant supplements such as curcumin, vitamin C, and astaxanthin. And remember, you're always beautiful—even more so as you gain wisdom with age.

Do you have sufficient vitamin D levels?

You know your body needs vitamin D, the sunshine vitamin, but were you aware that vitamin D is a steroid prohormone, which means the body converts vitamin D into a hormone? Only about 10 percent of our vitamin D comes from food. The rest comes from exposure to sunshine, which creates a chemical reaction in the skin, causing our bodies to make vitamin D, and is a primary source of this hormone. Vitamin D plays a significant role in graceful aging and overall health. For one, it helps the body absorb calcium, which helps with mineralization of bone that's necessary for strong bones.

Vitamin D deficiency causes a decrease in absorption of calcium and phosphorus from food. This can contribute to a decrease in bone mineral density, resulting in bone loss, osteopenia, and osteoporosis. In addition to its impact on bones, vitamin D influences many other parts of the body, including the intestines, the immune system, the cardiovascular system, the muscles, and the brain.

Low vitamin D has been associated with a wide range of health conditions, such as osteoporosis, muscle weakness, multiple sclerosis, depression, infections, heart disease, and diabetes.[145] Vitamin D helps regulate certain neurotransmitters, including serotonin, which helps explain its role in mood.[146] In women, low vitamin D has been linked to pregnancy problems, including preeclampsia (potentially life-threatening high blood pressure during pregnancy) and an increased need for cesarean section.[147]

People with darker skin tones need at least three to five times the length of sun exposure to make the same amount of vitamin D as someone with a pale complexion.[148] On top of this, aging itself causes our skin not to synthesize vitamin D as well.[149] Women are more at risk for vitamin D deficiency in the winter than in summer months, when we build up our stores.[150]

Getting your vitamin D levels tested is simple; your regular doctor can order it with routine blood work. Ask them to include 25-OH vitamin D during your next visit. I consider ideal levels to be on the upper end of the normal range (25–80 ng/mL).

Sleep and Stress

Do you get seven to eight hours of sleep each night and wake feeling rested?

No? It's okay, you're not alone. The good news is the seasonal reset program is perfect to help get you back on track with your sleep. For most people, seven to eight hours of uninterrupted sleep is ideal for obtaining the plethora of benefits and is what you want to aim for. Follow the mindset recommendations in the season you're in, and remember that certain times, such as during a full moon or a stressful day, can add extra challenges to sleep.[151] Let the changes with the sun be on your side—shift your activity level with it, setting your bedtime routine with the night's darkness each season. Sleep will likely be easier in the winter months, whereas summer nights may require more care for snoozing soundly.

Are you highly stressed more frequently than not?

If you're highly stressed, start incorporating daily mindset practices to help prevent cortisol from getting too high at night or too low in the morning. You may also want to consider taking adaptogenic herbs such as rhodiola and ashwagandha to help your body adjust and prevent health issues that can come from an imbalance of cortisol. Also, vitamin D_3 has been shown to help regulate different elements of both local and systemic HPA axes.[152]

Do you notice fatigue or mood changes in the fall and winter?

Yes? Then I recommend prioritizing mood-supportive practices in the summer to prepare for the cooler months ahead. Changes with light exposure can create disharmony with our chemical messengers related to energy, metabolism, and mood, so we want to shift our food, movement, and mindset accordingly. You may want to use light therapy in the fall and winter to help make up for the diminishing sunlight's benefits.

Do you have a history of physical or emotional trauma?

Many do, and if you're one of them, work with a well-trained therapist to get help unraveling emotional and physical symptoms that may be lingering. Trauma can impact your hormonal health, causing unpleasant symptoms, so it's important to get help.

Digestion and Detoxification

Do you experience digestive symptoms such as gas, bloating, heartburn, or abdominal discomfort?

If so, give your digestive system some love. Try adding 1 tablespoon of apple cider vinegar or lemon juice to a glass of water to drink before meals as a digestive aid. You may also want to consider taking a digestive enzyme before meals and a probiotic supplement. If you still have symptoms, talk to your healthcare provider about specialty lab testing to look for gut microbiome imbalances and other factors that may be impairing your digestion. Try to avoid taking antacids if you have heartburn because they increase the pH of your stomach, providing temporary relief but harming digestion in the long run because your stomach needs to be acidic for this process. Try to take antibiotics only when necessary as they can kill off the good bacteria in your body along with the bad bacteria.

Are you pooping regularly?

Ideally, we want to have bowel movements every day that are easy to pass and well formed. If you're not pooping every day or if it's difficult to pass, hard, broken, incomplete, soft, or runny, or contains undigested food particles, it's time to get your digestive system back on track. Follow the aforementioned digestion-supportive recommendations, and, if you're constipated, consider taking fiber, magnesium, or vitamin C supplements to help move things along. If those steps don't address your symptoms, consult your healthcare provider about testing and supplementation.

Are you currently or have you ever taken hormonal birth control, including birth control pills?

Birth control has changed our lives as women in a very profound way, helping us family plan around our productive lives. However, many girls and women are put on birth control pills for reasons other than birth control, including acne as well as menstrual irregularities and pain. But hormonal birth control pills contain synthetic forms of estrogen and progesterone and suppress our testosterone levels (impacting our sex drive and motivation), deplete us of certain nutrients, and disrupt our gut microbiota. And they come with a number of potential side effects, including an increased risk for blood clots, stroke, certain types of cancer (including breast, cervical, and uterine), and hormonal imbalances (such as low testosterone and low thyroid).

Unfortunately, I've seen too many women as patients who are working their way off or trying to reverse the damage caused by hormonal birth control. I had my own experience with these ill effects at age thirty, and I want to see you avoid these challenges. If you're looking for birth control, consider a nonhormonal form such as the copper IUD, or talk to your doctor about other options. If you're taking or have taken hormonal birth control, it's time to reverse the damage. Boost your nutrition and get your gut and detoxification back on track with the 7-Day Natural Beauty Reset for each season, and your hormonal balance will likely follow.

If you need extra help, work with a health-care provider who can test and lead you through a personalized program.

Are you highly sensitive or reactive to certain foods, skincare products, or chemicals?

I commonly see women who have numerous food, skincare, or chemical sensitivities also have leaky gut. When their gut lining is repaired, these sensitivities tend to go away or they're greatly diminished. To repair your gut lining, you may have a transition period when you'll need to be diligent about avoiding substances you're reactive to. Meanwhile, heal your gut lining with nourishing foods from this book and consider supplements like L-glutamine, aloe vera extract, marshmallow, N-acetyl-D-glucosamine (avoid if you have a shellfish allergy), and probiotics to soothe and repair your gut lining. If you need extra support, work with a naturopathic or functional medicine doctor.

Hormones

Are you experiencing any of the following symptoms: low sex drive, decreased sexual satisfaction, unexplained muscle wasting or bone loss, lack of motivation or drive, or prematurely thinning or sagging skin?

If you're facing these symptoms, and especially if you have more than a few of them, you may have low androgens (testosterone and DHEA). This often occurs with menopause, childbirth, adrenal stress, endometriosis, and taking birth control pills.[153]

If you suspect that's the case for you, get your levels tested. Following the 7-Day Natural Beauty Reset can help naturally support your androgen levels, especially when you exercise regularly, including performing weight-bearing exercises, and make dietary changes like consuming enough protein and healthy fats such as those from eggs, nuts, legumes, and wild salmon.

Because elevated cortisol levels can suppress testosterone, pay particular attention to the mindset practices and sleep recommendations in this book, and consider supplements like ashwagandha (250 to 500 mg) to help with de-stressing. Consider taking a vitamin D_3 supplement at around 3,000 IU daily, and if your 25-OH vitamin D levels are low-normal or low, bump that dose to 5,000 to 10,000 IU daily for a few months and then retest.[154]

Research suggests Tribulus[155] and zinc[156] supplements support healthy testosterone levels in women. Bioidentical hormones may provide additional support, and DHEA supplements are readily available, but it's important to start with a healthy lifestyle. Work with an experienced functional or naturopathic medicine doctor as hormones are intricately connected.

DHEA supplements may help support skin hydration and firmness, mood, and vaginal dryness. Although it's easy to get DHEA as a supplement at your local health food store, taking too much DHEA may cause issues such as moodiness, oily skin, acne, and facial hair growth.

Are you experiencing unwanted facial hair growth, hair loss on your scalp, infertility, menstrual irregularities, excessively oily or breakout-prone skin, higher sex drive, agitation, or anger than normal?

If you answer yes to any of these symptoms, you may have excess androgen levels. Touch base with your healthcare provider to test your hormone levels and determine if you have PCOS or other imbalances. If you're currently taking DHEA or testosterone, your doctor may need to lower your dosage. Within your seasonal eating plan, emphasize foods rich in zinc, and in the summertime, don't skimp on vitamin D—these can help balance testosterone and DHEA levels.

Chromium also appears to help lower free testosterone and is known for its blood sugar–balancing effects, two factors that are beneficial for women with PCOS. Saw palmetto is known for its ability to reduce androgen levels, such as in women with PCOS. Start with 160 mg daily. Melatonin[157] has been shown to help improve ovulation, particularly in women with PCOS.[158] High androgen levels suppress ovulation, and even if you're not actively trying to get pregnant, ovulation

is important for healthy hormonal balance, so you may want to consider taking melatonin at night.

Are you experiencing drier and inelastic skin, bone loss, hot flashes, night sweats, infertility, insomnia, mood changes, vaginal dryness, recurring UTIs or yeast infections, or urinary incontinence?

If you're having one or more of these symptoms, you may have low estrogen. Estrogen levels decline as we age, especially after forty, and our estrogen is also likely to be low before puberty, during high-stress times, just after pregnancy, and while breastfeeding. Women who have had their ovaries removed are in surgical menopause.

If you're having these symptoms, get your hormone levels tested to determine if your estrogen levels are low. You don't need to suffer through these symptoms and put yourself at higher risk for osteoporosis and cognitive decline, nor is it an ideal solution to take sleep medication or other pharmaceuticals that mask symptoms—you have alternative options. If you're just about to hit puberty, are breastfeeding, or are postpartum, talk with your doctor about ways to support your estrogen levels naturally and ease your way through this transition time naturally.

Eating certain phytoestrogens (naturally occurring plant compounds that are similar to estrogen in the human body) such as flaxseed, sesame seeds, non-GMO soy, and rhubarb may help support your estrogen levels naturally.[159] (Note: If you have a thyroid condition, you may want to limit your intake of certain phytoestrogens, such as soy, as they may interfere with thyroid function in susceptible individuals.)

Other lifestyle factors that appear to improve our estrogen levels include mindfulness approaches like yoga, as ongoing stress tends to suppress our estrogen production, including in young women.[160] And because oxytocin and estrogen[161] have a synergistic effect with each other, orgasms[162] and touch may help your estrogen levels.

You may want to take supplements like vitamin D_3, which has been shown to increase estrogen production.[163] Wild yams may help: women taking this wild veggie for thirty days saw an increase in estrogen and sex hormone–binding globulin levels, which attach to testosterone, DHT, and estrogen, and impact delivery amounts in the body.[164]

Melatonin is often deficient in postmenopausal women, so if you're at this stage, consider taking a melatonin supplement (start with 0.3 to 3.0 mg) at night.[165] Also, you can naturally support melatonin production with the sleep tips in this book. Additionally, taking curcumin (500 mg) and vitamin E (200 IU daily), two powerful antioxidants, has been shown to reduce hot flashes in postmenopausal women when taking for four weeks (curcumin) and eight weeks (vitamin E).[166]

Maca supplementation may help balance estrogen and progesterone, particularly in perimenopausal and postmenopausal women. Depending upon the source, 500 to 2,000 mg daily is often a good starting dose. With hot flashes, consider taking black cohosh because numerous studies have shown it to be helpful, especially during perimenopause and menopause.[167]

One of the ways many women address low estrogen is by using hormone replacement therapy. Throughout history, we've learned the hard way that synthetic estrogens (such as diethylstilbestrol [DES] and ethinyl estradiol) and Premarin (made from horse mare urine) are not molecularly similar to our own estrogens and can create harm in the body, so I recommend bioidentical forms.

Bioidentical estrogens typically are prescribed as estradiol and estriol, or a combination of the two. These are made in a lab from natural substances, and, when used properly and in combination with healthy lifestyle modifications, these and other bioidentical hormones can be a safe and effective way to help women make up for low hormones.

Have you experienced an early onset of your period, breast tenderness, irregular periods, weight gain, PMS/PMDD, irritability and mood swings before your period, cramping or painful periods, endometriosis, or migraine headaches during the second half of your cycle?

If you've experienced any of these symptoms, you may have high estrogen levels or what's often referred to as estrogen dominance, where estrogen is high in relation to progesterone. Women who are pregnant or on birth control pills generally have higher estrogen levels, and it's common for women over thirty-five to, at some point, experience symptoms of high estrogen dominance because progesterone levels usually drop before estrogen does as we get closer to menopause.

The key here is to help support healthy estrogen metabolism and ensure your hormones are balanced overall. This starts with following the 7-Day Natural Beauty Reset seasonal eating plan, including plenty of cruciferous vegetables, fiber, zinc-rich foods, high-antioxidant foods, and spices like turmeric.

There is evidence that light exposure impacts menstrual cycles due to the influence of melatonin, so we want to get a good night's sleep by following the movement and mindset practices to set us up for success.[168] And don't forget the importance of reducing exposures to EDCs in your environment and skincare. The Natural Beauty Reset program is your friend to turn to for help. From there, you can consider adding certain supplements to help enhance estrogen metabolism, support healthy detoxification pathways, plus balance estrogen and progesterone.

Taking 300 mg of diindolylmethane (DIM) daily is known for its ability to improve estrogen metabolism.[169] Turmeric has anti-inflammatory effects[170] and has been shown to reduce estradiol,[171] making this a great option for endometriosis and period pain. Zinc supplementation also appears to help decrease dysmenorrhea and endometriosis. Start with 15 mg twice daily for a few months and then talk to your healthcare provider about increasing your dose. Vitamin C and vitamin E are powerful antioxidants that have been shown to reduce the severity of dysmenorrhea.[172]

Are you experiencing irregular and/or heavy bleeding, fibroids, endometriosis, anxiousness, sadness, PMS/PMDD, hot flashes, night sweats, insomnia, or difficulty conceiving, or do you have a history of multiple miscarriages?

If you have one or more of these symptoms, you may have low progesterone. Perimenopausal symptoms can start around age thirty-five, when a drop in progesterone often occurs. If you can, ask your mom when she went through menopause, as your experience may mirror hers given that the timing and symptoms of menopause have a strong genetic component. Knowing the answer can help you plan ahead for hormonal changes.

As with other hormones, balance is key, so following the Natural Beauty Reset program's food, movement, and mindset practices can help support your body's natural ability to produce progesterone in balance with other hormones.

Some recommendations to boost progesterone in relation to estrogen include taking 500 to 1,000 mg of chasteberry (also known as vitex) daily. Chasteberry can support progesterone levels and reduce PMS/PMDD. Melatonin has been shown to improve the production of progesterone, too.[173] And GLA, such as in evening primrose oil (starting at 500 mg once to twice daily), has been shown to help reduce breast tenderness, PMS, and hot flashes.[174] Consuming 750 mg of vitamin C daily has been shown to help increase progesterone.[175]

Bioidentical progesterone hormone replacement therapy is used to help women with low progesterone maintain a healthy pregnancy and minimize symptoms during perimenopause. I personally love this hormone because of its mood-boosting and sleep-promoting benefits, and taking progesterone helped me achieve a healthy pregnancy after a miscarriage at age thirty-two. And I'm not alone. Many of my patients and other women have benefited from the use of progesterone as part of a holistic treatment program.

Progestin, which is found in oral contraceptives, hormonal IUDs, and hormone replacement therapy, is the synthetic form of progesterone. While many women are prescribed this form, there are concerns, some of which arose in the Women's Health Initiative (WHI) study. Side effects observed in some of those participants ranged from abnormal periods, blood clots, heart attacks, and strokes to depression, skin rashes, migraines, and liver problems. Because of these potential risk factors, I recommend women stick with bioidentical progesterone.

The bottom line is to always start with lifestyle adjustments and then add in supplements such as chasteberry. If that's not enough, then find an integrative healthcare provider specializing in women's hormones who can help you with the right dose of bioidentical hormones, monitor your progress, and make adjustments as needed. Optimizing progesterone levels will mean a brighter mood, better sleep, and potentially improved fertility, among other results that will help you inch closer toward realizing your natural beauty.

Are you using hormone replacement therapy?

If so, talk with your healthcare provider about a bioidentical version, if you're not already on one.

The WHI trials in 1991 looked at hormonal therapies including Premarin and progestin, and the scientists stopped the study after observing an increased risk of heart disease, stroke, blood clots, and breast cancer in participants. Since this study was halted in 2002, we've learned a lot more about hormonal therapies and the difference between synthetic and natural forms of certain hormones, as well as those that are bioidentical. Bioidentical hormones are molecularly the same as our natural hormones, so our bodies have an easier time discerning how to properly use and metabolize them.

I've been prescribing bioidentical hormones to patients for over twenty years and have found them to help manage symptoms during certain transition times, such as perimenopause, and help protect against common concerns for women over fifty, including bone loss.

If you're using hormone replacement therapy, get your hormone levels (including their metabolites) tested regularly. For my patients, I order a combination of urine, salivary, and blood tests. Follow the food recommendations for each season, and ensure that your detoxification and digestive systems are working optimally to help your chances for proper hormone metabolism. Also, review the chapter on hormones so you understand how your hormones work and can identify when yours may be imbalanced.

Do you experience fatigue (especially in the mornings), dizziness (especially when standing up), low blood pressure, weight loss, or muscle weakness?

If you experience some of these symptoms, your adrenal glands may be struggling to produce optimal levels of cortisol. While cortisol often gets a bad rap, it's a helpful hormone in our daily lives, helping us wake up in the morning and appropriately respond to stressful situations. If you have

these symptoms, check with your healthcare provider about getting your cortisol levels tested with multiple salivary or urine collections made throughout a day. Addison's disease is a potentially life-threatening form of low cortisol and is more severe than suboptimal adrenal function, so if you have this condition or suspect you may, talk with your doctor about testing and treatment.

Lifestyle factors are essential for balancing adrenal function, so pay particular attention to the mindset practices for each season. You can also consider supplements such as adaptogenic herbs (rhodiola or ashwagandha), B vitamin complex, vitamin C, and licorice root extract (avoid if you have high blood pressure).

Do you have issues with insomnia, excess belly fat, sugar cravings, or inflammatory skin conditions like acne, eczema, or rosacea?

If you experience some or all of these symptoms, your adrenal glands may be producing higher than normal levels of cortisol, which could either be ongoing or more focused in the later hours of the day, which is the opposite of healthy adrenal function.

To help balance adrenal function, focus on healthy eating, movement, and mindset practices from the 7-Day Natural Beauty Reset. In addition, consider taking some of the following supplements to help balance your cortisol levels: phosphatidylserine, L-theanine, L-tyrosine, Panax ginseng, ashwagandha, or rhodiola. The dosing on these can vary, depending on the complexity of your health issues and the level at which your adrenals are functioning.

Do you have fatigue, constipation, hair loss, weight gain, irregular menses, infertility, or dry, coarse skin with a reduced ability to perspire?

If you have at least a few of these symptoms, you may have low or suboptimal thyroid hormone levels. Hypothyroidism is a common hormonal imbalance in women that often goes undiagnosed for many years. When testing your thyroid levels, ask your doctor to run a full panel and include thyroid antibodies. Review the chapter on hormones to understand more about the thyroid.

Because the thyroid is necessary for proper metabolism, pay particular attention to food and movement. Also, reduce exposures to EDCs and tame stress through mindset practices because adrenal and thyroid function are closely interconnected. Zinc, selenium, iodine, and tyrosine support your thyroid function, so eat foods with these and discuss supplements with your functional medicine or naturopathic doctor.[176]

Also ask your doctor if you're a good candidate for natural desiccated thyroid or other thyroid medication. With my patients, I typically prescribe a combination of T3 and T4 for optimal thyroid support in addition to my Natural Beauty Reset program and certain supplements, such as zinc, selenium, and N-acetyl-L-tyrosine.

If you have an autoimmune thyroid condition (high thyroid antibodies), focus on balancing your immune system while you're supporting thyroid function. You'll want to address your gut and work with a naturopathic or functional medicine doctor who can help you restore overall hormonal balance on your journey toward achieving natural beauty.

Do you experience warm, sweaty, and flushed skin, feel overstimulated, have diarrhea or loose stools, or have difficulty keeping weight on?

If you're experiencing some or all of these symptoms, you may have hyperthyroidism. Request thyroid level testing to find out, and ask your doctor for a full thyroid panel and thyroid antibodies. This can help catch early signs of thyroid imbalance as well as help monitor your levels. Remember, there are solutions to hormonal imbalances, and you're the CEO of your health, so be proactive instead of reactive when you have symptoms or receive a diagnosis.

Do you experience increased thirst and appetite, tingling sensations in your hands and feet, fatigue, irritability, headaches, PCOS, or frequent urination or infections?

If you answered yes to any or all of those symptoms, you may have insulin resistance, or difficulty with balancing your blood sugar. Insulin resistance can also cause imbalances in estrogen and progesterone levels, and can trigger PCOS.[177] Ask your healthcare provider for testing to determine if you have optimal glucose and insulin levels, and review the hormones chapter to learn more about insulin resistance.

Each season, pay attention to blood sugar regulation by eating balanced meals containing fiber, protein, and healthy fats, and minimizing foods that spike your blood sugar such as high-carbohydrate foods and those containing sugar and HFCS. You'll notice, in this book, the recipes contain only minimal amounts of sweeteners, which is important to help stay on track. You may choose to replace honey and maple syrup with stevia, monk fruit, or erythritol because these alternatives do not increase blood sugar. Also, keep your cortisol levels balanced with the mindset and movement practices in this book, and reduce your exposures to EDCs.

Do you see your healthcare provider regularly?

If you have health concerns or haven't seen your doctor within the last year, I encourage you to schedule an appointment to discuss any symptoms you have, get a checkup, and run some lab tests to make sure your hormones and overall health is well balanced. Be mindful of who you choose to manage your healthcare and be sure they're on the same page as you. Your body is yours alone and you're the boss. Your primary healthcare provider and healthcare team should respect your decision-making abilities. Most conventionally trained doctors do not have the training for nutritional and herbal supplements, nor will they know to instinctively order specialty lab tests mentioned in this book, so if you want help with addressing root causes such as hormonal imbalances, nutritional deficiencies, and gut microbiota issues using an integrative/holistic approach, work with a licensed naturopathic doctor or functional medicine doctor (see resources at the end of this book).

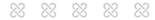

Pulling it all together . . .

Your body is wise and simply needs the right tools to restore harmony. With the answers to the questions in this chapter, you're able to follow the 7-Day Natural Beauty Reset with a more customized approach. This means you have the ability to address underlying imbalances and lifestyle factors so you can have that natural glow—the kind that turns heads—while inside you feel energized and resilient. You're able to optimize your superpowers as a woman because you're balanced and have a body that bounces back, just as it was designed to do. And as you stand in your authentic radiance in front of the mirror, remember: your beauty was always there. Now, it's just easier to see.

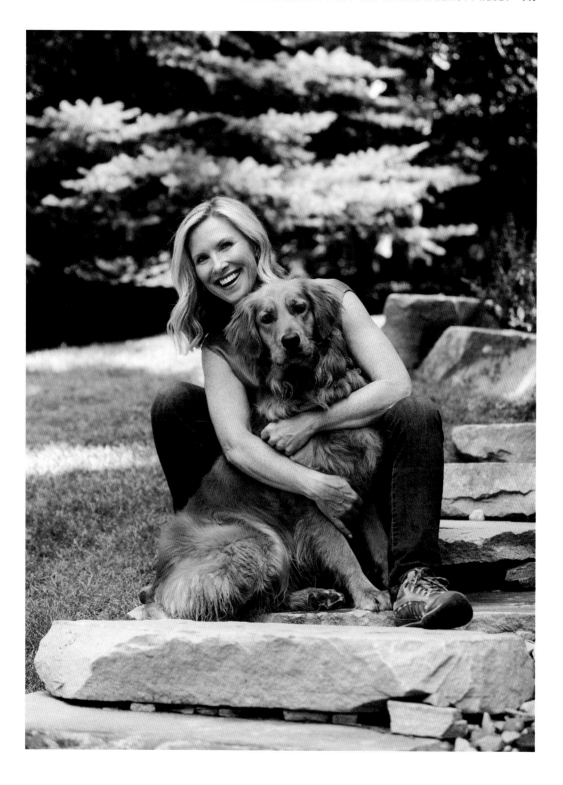

CHAPTER 13

NATURAL BEAUTY RESET RECIPES

FOOD RECIPES

You'll find seventy-six healthy and delicious food recipes in this section. Every season includes options for breakfast, lunch and dinner, and snacks and desserts. Enjoy!

FALL RECIPES

BREAKFAST

Pumpkin Spice Smoothie

Bring in the fall flavors of pumpkin, cinnamon, and ginger in the form of a nourishing smoothie. Pumpkin is rich in the antioxidant beta carotene, cinnamon helps balance blood sugar, and ginger aids digestion. The perfect combination for a fall reset!

SERVES 1 | PREP TIME: 5 MINUTES

- ½ cup unsweetened pumpkin purée
- 1 cup organic unsweetened vanilla almond or hazelnut milk
- ½ cup ice (optional)
- 1 tablespoon almond butter or ¼ cup raw almonds, soaked

- ½ teaspoon cinnamon
- ¼ teaspoon peeled and grated fresh ginger, or dried ginger
- 2 pitted Medjool dates, soaked for 10 minutes in hot water to soften for easier blending (soaking optional)

In a blender, combine the pumpkin purée, milk, ice (if using), almond butter, cinnamon, ginger, and dates, and blend until smooth. Pour into a tall glass and enjoy.

Tip for a thicker consistency: Freeze half of the almond milk into ice cubes before blending. If choosing this option, eliminate ice cubes from ingredients.

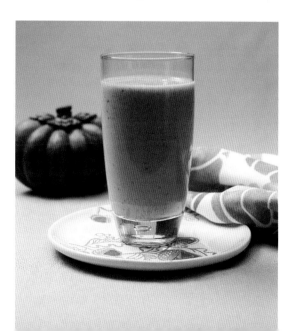

Ginger Chia Pudding with Pomegranate Seeds

Pudding for breakfast? Yes! When it's this healthy, you can easily splurge for breakfast. Start your fall morning with warming ginger and a burst of flavor from antioxidant-rich pomegranate seeds.

SERVES 3 TO 4 | PREP TIME: 5 MINUTES, PLUS 20 MINUTES FOR THICKENING

- 2 cups organic unsweetened almond milk
- 3 pitted dates, soaked in hot water for 10 minutes to soften
- ½ cup raw pecans
- ½ teaspoon pure vanilla extract
- ½ teaspoon peeled and grated fresh ginger, or ½ teaspoon dried ginger
- Pinch sea salt
- ½ cup chia seeds
- ¼ cup pomegranate seeds

In a high-speed blender, combine the almond milk, dates, pecans, vanilla, ginger, and salt. Blend until creamy and smooth. Place the chia seeds in a medium bowl, pour the blended ingredients over the chia seeds, and stir well to combine. Let sit for at least 20 minutes or until the pudding thickens. Serve at room temperature or refrigerate and serve cold. Top with pomegranate seeds.

Overnight Chia Oats

Get a boost of fiber with oats and chia seeds to help balance blood sugar and hormones. Top with fresh fall fruit like apples, pears, or figs. You can also make this the night before for a nourishing breakfast on the go.

SERVES 2 | PREP TIME: 5 MINUTES, PLUS OVERNIGHT REFRIGERATION

- 1 cup old-fashioned rolled oats
- 2 tablespoons chia seeds
- 2 cups unsweetened almond or hazelnut milk
- ½ teaspoon ground cinnamon
- 2 to 4 teaspoons raw honey (to taste)
- ½ cup chopped apples, pears, or fresh figs

Mix the oats, chia seeds, milk, cinnamon, and honey together in a large mason jar. Let sit in the refrigerator overnight. In the morning, serve cool or heat up to warm. Top with fruit before serving.

Ultimate Green Smoothie Juice

Even while the leaves are turning to shades of yellow, orange, and red, you can get a green burst with this ultimate smoothie. It's light like a juice but packed full of fiber and antioxidants. Fresh and delicious, the flavors meld for a healthy fall treat. The ginger tea pairs deliciously with the sourness of the grapes and apple.

SERVES 1 | PREP TIME: 5 MINUTES

- ½ cup frozen green grapes
- 1 tablespoon spirulina
- 1 cup chopped organic kale, packed
- 1 cup chilled, unsweetened ginger tea
- 2 teaspoons chia seeds
- ¼ medium green apple
- ½ lemon, juiced (optional)

In a blender, combine the grapes, spirulina, kale, ginger tea, chia seeds, green apple, and lemon juice (if using), and blend until smooth. Pour into a tall glass, chill in the refrigerator to desired temperature, and enjoy.

LUNCH AND DINNER

Halibut Tacos with Red Cabbage Slaw

Brighten up your fall days with this colorful, flavorful recipe. Fresh halibut is easier to find this time of year, and paired with ripe peppers and red cabbage, it allows you to savor the tastes of fall.

SERVES 3 TO 4 | PREP TIME: 20 MINUTES | COOK TIME: 15 MINUTES

RED CABBAGE SLAW:

- 3 tablespoons red onion, diced
- 1 cup shredded purple cabbage
- ½ cup stemmed, seeded, and diced red, orange, or yellow bell peppers
- 1 tablespoon lime juice
- 1 tablespoon avocado oil
- 2 cloves garlic, minced
- 2 tablespoons chopped fresh cilantro
- Sea salt to taste

HALIBUT TACOS:

- 10 to 12 small collard greens leaves, thick stem trimmed
- ½ teaspoon sea salt
- 2 teaspoons garlic powder
- 1 teaspoon onion powder
- ¼ teaspoon chili powder
- 4 (4- to 5-ounce) skinless halibut fillets, cut into two to three pieces each
- 2 to 3 tablespoons avocado oil
- Lime wedges, for garnish

FOR THE SLAW:

In a medium bowl, combine the red onion, purple cabbage, bell pepper, lime juice, avocado oil, garlic, and cilantro, and mix to combine.

FOR THE TACOS:

In a large saucepan, heat water to a boil over high heat. Prepare an ice bath of water to the side of the stove. Carefully blanch the collard greens leaves for 10 seconds in the boiling water until bright green and softened. Immediately place the leaves into the ice water to stop the cooking process. Once cool, move to a paper towel and pat dry.

Combine the salt, garlic powder, onion powder, and chili powder in a small bowl. Season the fish pieces on both sides by dipping it in the bowl until well coated.

In a large skillet over medium-high heat, heat the avocado oil. Carefully place the fillets in the pan. Cook for 2 to 3 minutes on each side, carefully flipping, until the fish is opaque and easily flakes with a fork.

Place one piece of fish on a collard greens leaf, top with the slaw, and fold the collard greens leaf like a taco. Serve with a lime wedge and repeat with the remaining ingredients.

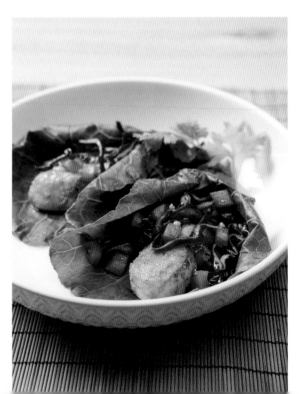

Turkey Meatballs with Parsley Pesto and Zucchini Pasta

Fall is the time of turkey and zucchini, so we bring them together in this zesty dish. Grab a veggie spiralizer and enjoy the fall harvest with fresh herb pesto packed full of nutrients that nourish your body and soul.

SERVES 5 TO 6 (5 CUPS NOODLES, 20 MEATBALLS, 1 CUP PESTO)
PREP TIME: 20 MINUTES | COOK TIME: 15 MINUTES

TURKEY MEATBALLS:
- 1 pound ground free-range turkey
- 1 tablespoon chia seeds
- 1 tablespoon chopped garlic
- ½ tablespoon whole-grain mustard
- ½ tablespoon dried parsley
- ½ tablespoon dried oregano
- ½ tablespoon dried sage
- ½ tablespoon onion powder
- ½ teaspoon salt
- 2 slices gluten-free bread, torn apart into small pieces
- Avocado oil cooking spray

PARSLEY PESTO:
- ½ cup pine nuts
- 2 cups fresh parsley, packed
- 3 garlic cloves
- ½ teaspoon sea salt
- ½ lemon, juiced
- ½ cup extra-virgin olive oil

ZUCCHINI PASTA:
- 2 (8-ounce) medium zucchini
- 2 (8-ounce) medium yellow squash
- 1 tablespoon avocado oil (optional)

FOR THE MEATBALLS:

Preheat the oven to 400°F. Line two baking sheets with parchment paper.

Combine the turkey, chia seeds, garlic, mustard, parsley, oregano, sage, onion powder, salt, and gluten-free bread. Form into meatballs about 1.5 inches in diameter and place on the prepared baking sheets. Spray with avocado oil cooking spray and bake for 12 minutes or until a meat thermometer registers 165°F.

FOR THE PESTO:

Add the pine nuts, parsley, garlic, salt, and lemon juice to the bowl of a food processor. Pulse until finely chopped. While the machine is running, slowly drizzle in the olive oil and pulse until smooth and combined.

FOR THE PASTA:

Using a spiralizer, spiralize the zucchini and yellow squash into "noodles."

For cooked noodles, heat a large sauté pan with 1 tablespoon avocado oil over medium-high heat. Add the zucchini and squash noodles and cook for 1 to 2 minutes until warm but still al dente. Season with salt and pepper.

Serve the meatballs over uncooked or cooked spiralized zucchini and yellow squash, and top with pesto.

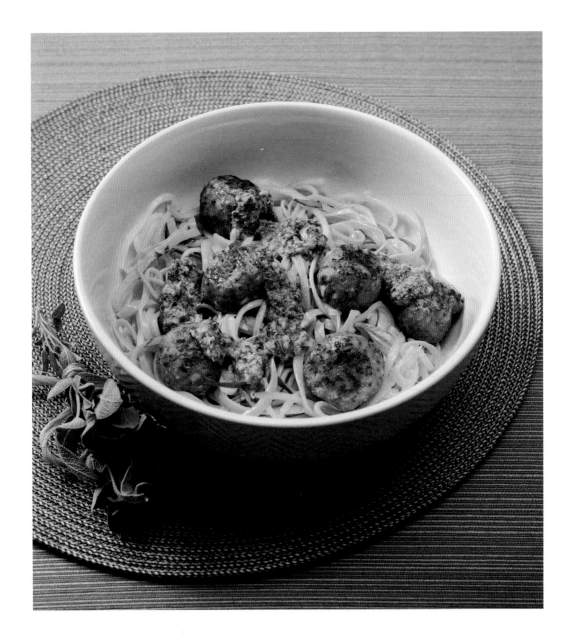

White Bean Soup with Collard Greens

I like to enjoy this soup by the fire at the end of my day. It's so warm and comforting with plenty of protein (despite not having meat), herbs that indulge the palate, and almonds that add a crunch.

SERVES 4 TO 5 | PREP TIME: 10 MINUTES | COOK TIME: 35 MINUTES

- 1 tablespoon coconut oil
- 1 small white onion, chopped
- 2 carrots, peeled and chopped
- 4 cloves garlic, minced
- 1 tablespoon dried thyme
- 1 teaspoon dried oregano
- 1 teaspoon dried sage
- 1 teaspoon sea salt
- ¼ teaspoon freshly ground black pepper

- 1 cup dry cannellini beans, cooked (3 cups when cooked) or 2 (15-ounce) cans cannellini beans, drained and rinsed
- 4 cups vegetable or chicken broth
- 2 cups chopped collard greens or kale
- 1 lemon, juiced for garnish
- ½ cup chopped raw almonds for garnish
- 2 tablespoons extra-virgin olive oil for garnish
- 2 tablespoons chopped fresh parsley for garnish

Heat the coconut oil in a large Dutch oven or pot over medium-high heat. Add the onion, carrots, and garlic, and cook for 3 to 4 minutes until softened. Add the thyme, oregano, sage, salt, and pepper, and cook for another 30 seconds until aromatic.

Add the beans and broth. Bring to a boil, then reduce to a simmer. Allow to simmer for 25 to 30 minutes until flavors blend and meld together. During the last 10 minutes of cooking, stir in the collard greens and simmer until tender. Stir in the lemon juice.

Divide among bowls and garnish with almonds, olive oil, and fresh parsley.

Quinoa Lentil Salad with Roasted Eggplant

As the cooler weather sets in, this recipe will give you a healthy dose of vitamins A and C from eggplant and fiber fuel from quinoa and lentils—all mixed in with a tasty dressing topped with toasted pumpkin seeds to provide a satisfying crunch.

SERVES 5 TO 6 | PREP TIME: 30 MINUTES | COOK TIME: 30 MINUTES

ROASTED EGGPLANT:
- 1 (1½-pound) eggplant, peeled and diced into ¾-inch cubes (about 7.5 cups)
- ¼ cup avocado oil
- ½ teaspoon sea salt

QUINOA LENTIL SALAD:
- ⅓ cup raw pumpkin seeds, toasted
- 1 cup green lentils, rinsed
- 2 cups quinoa, rinsed
- ⅓ cup extra-virgin olive oil
- ⅓ cup apple cider vinegar
- 2 teaspoon Dijon mustard
- 2 cloves garlic, minced
- 1 teaspoon sea salt
- Ground black pepper to taste
- 2 ribs celery, thinly sliced (1 cup)
- 5 small carrots, peeled and thinly sliced (1 cup)
- ½ head fennel, cored and chopped (1 cup)
- ¼ cup chopped parsley

FOR THE ROASTED EGGPLANT:

Preheat the oven to 350°F. Line two baking sheets with parchment paper.

Divide the eggplant evenly between the two baking sheets, toss in ¼ cup avocado oil, and season with salt. Roast for 30 minutes, flipping halfway through, until golden brown and tender. Allow to cool.

FOR THE QUINOA LENTIL SALAD:

To toast the pumpkin seeds, place a small sauté pan over medium-low heat and add the pumpkin seeds. Allow to toast until golden and fragrant, 3 to 5 minutes. Move to a bowl and allow to cool.

Meanwhile, in a large pot, bring about 6 cups of water to a boil. Add the lentils, return to a boil, then reduce to low, cover, and simmer for 15 minutes until the lentils are starting to soften. Add the quinoa and cook together for an additional 10 to 15 minutes until the lentils are tender and the quinoa is fully cooked. Strain, rinse with cold water, and set aside.

In a large bowl, whisk together the olive oil, vinegar, mustard, garlic, salt, and pepper. Add the celery, carrots, fennel, cooled quinoa and lentils, pumpkin seeds, and parsley. Toss to evenly coat. Top with the eggplant and serve. Season with additional salt if desired.

This salad can be served warm, room temperature, or chilled. It stores well in an airtight container in the fridge for up to four days.

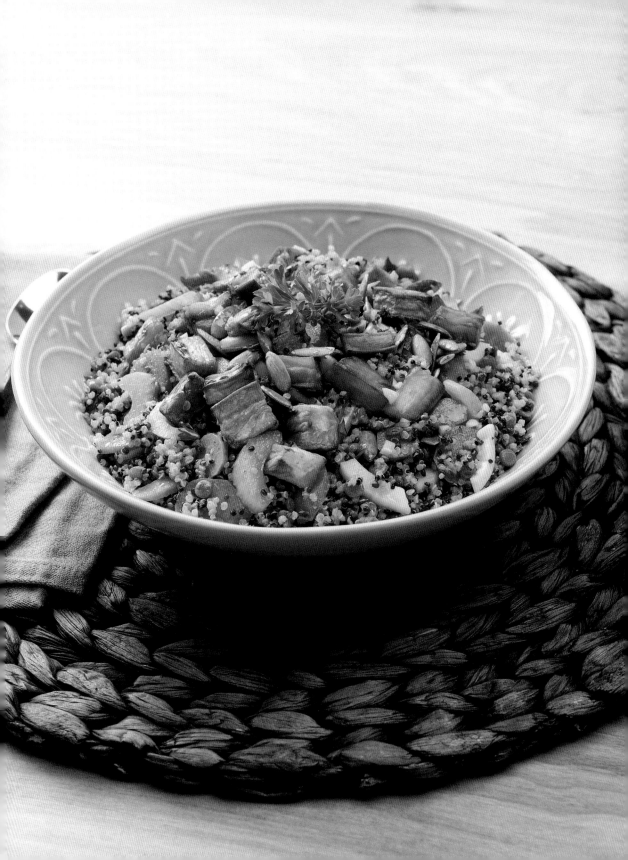

Lime Chili Halibut with Garlic Kale

Zest up your fall with this lime- and chili-flavored fish dish. Kale, in full nutrient-dense season, is tender, and the garlic gives it an extra kick.

SERVES 3 TO 4 (4 FILLETS AND 6 CUPS KALE) | PREP TIME: 15 MINUTES, PLUS 1 HOUR FOR MARINATING | COOK TIME: 15 MINUTES

LIME CHILI HALIBUT:

- 4 tablespoons lime juice
- 2 tablespoons avocado oil
- ½ tablespoon chili powder
- 3 cloves garlic, crushed
- 1 teaspoon sea salt
- 4 fillets (about 2 pounds) skinless halibut, about 1-inch thick
- Lime wedges, to serve

GARLIC KALE:

- 3 tablespoons avocado oil
- 1 small yellow onion, diced
- 6 cloves garlic, crushed or chopped
- 2 bunches curly kale (about 1 pound), destemmed and chopped (about 19 cups chopped)
- ½ teaspoon sea salt , plus additional to taste
- ¼ cup vegetable broth or water
- Freshly ground black pepper to taste

FOR THE LIME CHILI HALIBUT:

Combine the lime juice, avocado oil, chili powder, garlic, and salt in a shallow baking dish. Add the halibut steaks in a single layer and turn a few times to coat the fish. Cover and allow to marinate in the refrigerator for about an hour.

Preheat the grill to high heat or the oven to 400°F. If using the oven, line a baking sheet with parchment paper.

Grill or bake the halibut fillets for about 4 to 5 minutes per side, until the fish is opaque and flakes easily with a fork. If roasting the fish, drain the fillets of excess marinade and place them on the prepared baking sheet. Roast them for about 12 to 14 minutes or until opaque and the fish flakes easily with a fork.

FOR THE GARLIC KALE:

Heat the oil in a large pot over medium-high heat. When the oil is warm, add the onion and garlic. Sauté until the onion is translucent, 3 to 4 minutes. Add the kale, season with salt, and sauté until tender, about 4 to 5 minutes. Add the broth or water and allow it to cook another 2 to 4 minutes, until the kale is wilted and tender. Season with additional salt and pepper to taste.

Serve the fillets over the garlic kale with a lime wedge for garnish.

Creamy Broccoli Soup

Craving creamy comfort food? Here's a flavorful, creamy soup without any real cream. You won't even realize how healthy you're eating since the beans provide richness and creaminess when blended with broccoli.

SERVES 3 TO 4 | PREP TIME: 15 MINUTES | COOK TIME: 30 MINUTES

- 1 tablespoon avocado oil
- 1 small yellow onion, diced
- 3 cloves garlic, minced or crushed
- 1 teaspoon fresh thyme leaves
- ½ teaspoon sea salt, plus additional to taste
- 4 cups broccoli florets (from two heads of broccoli, about 1 pound)
- 1 cup diced red or Yukon Gold potatoes
- 1 rib of celery, chopped
- 1½ cups cooked white beans or 1 (15-ounce) can cannellini beans, drained and rinsed
- 4 cups vegetable or free-range chicken broth
- 1 cup full-fat coconut milk, well-shaken

Heat a large pot with avocado oil over medium-high heat. Add the onion and garlic and sauté until the onion is translucent, 3 to 4 minutes. Add the thyme and season with salt.

Add the broccoli, potatoes, celery, white beans, and vegetable broth. Bring to a boil, then reduce to a simmer. Allow to simmer for 10 to 15 minutes or until the broccoli florets and potatoes are very tender.

Transfer the soup in batches to the carafe of a high-speed blender. Blend until very smooth and return the soup to the pot. Add the coconut milk and stir to combine. Season with additional salt as needed and serve.

Black Bean Turkey Chili

Looking for something hearty to counterbalance cooler temperatures? Warm up with this seasonal fiber-filled chili. Since black beans have more antioxidants than any other bean, you'll find this recipe is rich in nutrients in addition to flavor.

SERVES 3 TO 4 | PREP TIME: 15 MINUTES | COOK TIME: 45 MINUTES

- 1 tablespoon avocado oil
- 1 small yellow onion, chopped
- 1 red bell pepper, stemmed, seeded, and diced
- 2 to 3 cloves garlic, minced
- 1 pound ground free-range turkey
- 1 teaspoon sea salt, plus additional to taste
- 3 tablespoons chili powder
- 1 teaspoon dried oregano
- 1 (15-ounce) can chopped tomatoes
- 3 to 4 cups chicken stock
- 2 cups cooked or 1 (15-ounce) can black beans, drained and rinsed
- 2 scallions, thinly sliced for garnish

Heat a large Dutch oven or pot over medium-high heat with avocado oil. Add the onion, bell pepper, and garlic, and cook until softened, 4 to 5 minutes. Add the ground turkey and season with salt. Allow the turkey to cook until browned, breaking it into pieces using the back of a wooden spoon, 7 to 9 minutes.

During the last minute of the turkey cooking, add the chili powder and oregano. Allow the spices to toast for a minute, coating the meat, then add the tomatoes, stock, and beans, and bring to a boil. Reduce to a simmer and allow to simmer for 20 to 30 minutes (if you have time, feel free to simmer longer!). Season with additional salt as needed and serve. Garnish with thinly sliced scallions.

Red Lentil Soup

These delicious and tender lentils with turmeric, ginger, and fennel will spice up your day. And you'll receive the anti-inflammatory benefits of these herbs and spices with an extra nourishment from spinach stirred in as a nice fresh boost at the end.

SERVES 2 TO 3 │ PREP TIME: 5 MINUTES, PLUS 1 TO 3 HOURS FOR SOAKING
COOK TIME: 45 MINUTES

- 1 cup red lentils
- 4 teaspoons ghee or coconut oil
- 2 cloves garlic, minced
- ½ teaspoon ground ginger
- ½ teaspoon ground turmeric
- 1 teaspoon ground fennel
- 1 teaspoon ground coriander
- 1 teaspoon ground cumin
- 1 teaspoon sea salt
- ½ teaspoon freshly ground black pepper
- 4 cups vegetable or free-range chicken broth
- 2 cups baby spinach leaves

If time allows, soak the lentils for 1 to 3 hours prior to cooking. Wash and drain the lentils.

In a medium-size pot, heat the ghee over medium heat. Add the garlic, ginger, turmeric, fennel, coriander, and cumin, and allow to toast for a minute until fragrant. Add the lentils and stir to coat with the spices. Season with salt and pepper. Add the broth, and bring to a boil.

Cover with a lid and reduce the heat to low. Allow to simmer for 35 minutes until the lentils are very tender. During the last 5 minutes of cooking, stir in the spinach, and allow it to wilt.

Roasted Brussels Sprouts and Apple Salad

Relish fall flavors with this salad topped with warm and delicious apples and brussels sprouts with a light sweetness from raw honey and pomegranate seeds. It's so naturally colorful, which means antioxidants abound!

SERVES 2 TO 3 | PREP TIME: 15 MINUTES | COOK TIME: 28 MINUTES

DRESSING:
- ¼ cup extra-virgin olive oil
- ¼ cup fresh lemon juice
- 1 tablespoon raw honey
- 1 teaspoon Dijon mustard
- Sea salt and freshly ground black pepper to taste

ROASTED BRUSSELS SPROUTS
AND APPLE SALAD:
- 2 cups (8 ounces) cleaned, trimmed, and halved brussels sprouts
- 1 organic red apple (such as honey crisp), peeled, cored, and sliced ¼-inch thick
- 1 tablespoon coconut oil
- ½ teaspoon sea salt
- 1 teaspoon fresh thyme
- 5 ounces baby spinach
- ½ cup toasted and chopped almonds or walnut halves
- ¼ cup pomegranate seeds

FOR THE DRESSING:

In a medium bowl whisk together the olive oil, lemon juice, honey, and mustard until combined. Season with salt and pepper and set aside.

FOR THE ROASTED BRUSSELS SPROUTS AND APPLE SALAD:

Preheat the oven to 375°F. Line a baking sheet with parchment paper.

In a large bowl, toss the brussels sprouts, apple, oil, salt, and thyme together. Place the brussels sprouts mixture evenly onto the prepared baking sheet. Roast uncovered for 25 to 28 minutes, flipping the brussels sprouts and apples halfway through, until golden brown and tender.

Serve the roasted brussels sprouts mixture over a bed of fresh baby spinach. Garnish with nuts and pomegranate seeds, and drizzle with dressing.

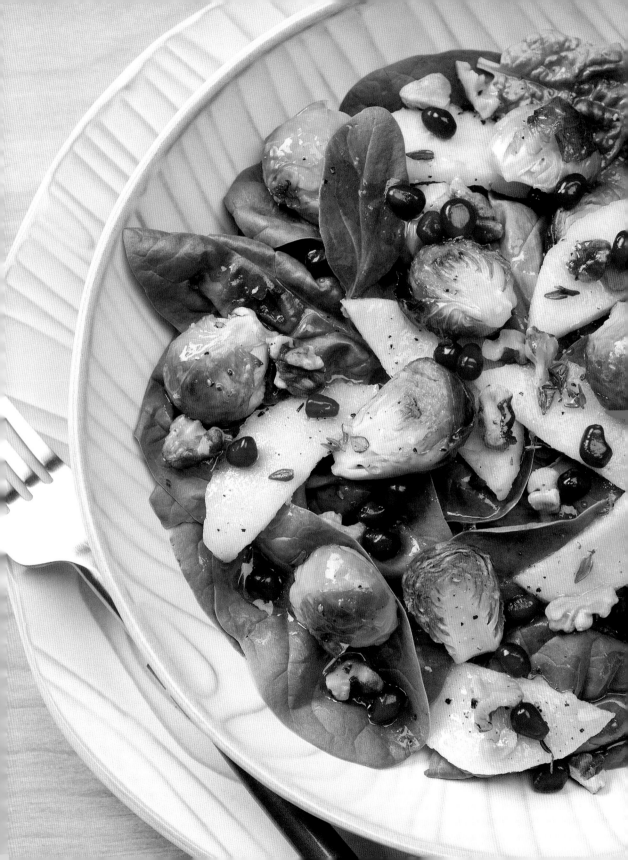

Fall Harvest Salad

Fall harvest is full of dark, rich colors, and this salad is the perfect representation with nice earthy flavors from beets and chickpeas. This is a filling and balanced combination of fall flavors and nutrients.

SERVES 2 TO 3 | PREP TIME: 20 MINUTES

DRESSING:
- ¼ cup extra-virgin olive oil
- 2 tablespoons apple cider vinegar
- 1 tablespoon chopped fresh rosemary
- 1 tablespoon chopped fresh thyme
- 1 teaspoon Dijon mustard
- ½ teaspoon sea salt
- ¼ teaspoon freshly ground black pepper

SALAD:
- 1 (5-ounce) container mix of baby kale, spinach, or frisée
- 1 cup chopped red cabbage
- 1 carrot, peeled and thinly sliced
- 1 medium beet, peeled and shredded
- 4 red radishes, chopped
- ½ cup chopped pecans
- 1 (15-ounce) can garbanzo beans, drained and rinsed

FOR THE DRESSING:

In a small bowl, whisk the olive oil, vinegar, rosemary, thyme, and mustard together until well combined. Season to taste with salt and pepper.

FOR THE SALAD:

In a large bowl, add the greens, cabbage, carrot, beet, radishes, pecans, and garbanzo beans. Drizzle the dressing around the rim of the bowl and toss together until well combined.

Beau Pa's Cookies

My father would be proud to see his cookies here. He's no longer with us, but his legendary cookies live on. Though he never followed a recipe, my daughter Thalia and I came up with a recipe I think he'd be happy to see! This is the perfect chewy treat with fall-focused spices and dried fruit for extra sweetness. With no sugar added and full of fiber, these treats are ones you can give in to the craving for more than one.

1 DOZEN COOKIES | SERVES 4 TO 6 | PREP TIME: 15 MINUTES | COOK TIME: 12 MINUTES

- ¼ cup unsalted grass-fed butter or organic coconut oil
- ¼ cup raw honey
- 1 tablespoon unsweetened plain almond milk
- 3 tablespoons unsweetened applesauce
- 1 teaspoon vanilla
- 1 cup gluten-free flour (equal parts tapioca, coconut, and rice flours)
- ½ teaspoon baking soda
- 1 teaspoon xanthan gum
- ½ teaspoon ground or fresh ginger
- 1 teaspoon cinnamon
- ½ teaspoon sea salt
- ½ cup gluten-free rolled oats
- 2 tablespoons chopped walnuts
- 2 tablespoons raisins

Preheat the oven to 350°F. Line a baking sheet with parchment paper.

In a large bowl using a hand mixer, or in the bowl of a stand mixer fitted with the paddle attachment, beat the butter and honey together until smooth. Add the almond milk, applesauce, and vanilla, and beat again.

Add the flour, baking soda, xanthan gum, ginger, cinnamon, and sea salt. Stir in the oats, walnuts, and raisins. Scoop the dough into 2 tablespoon-size balls and place them on the prepared baking sheet about 2 inches apart from one another. Gently press down on the dough to flatten. Bake for 12 minutes until golden brown. Allow to cool on the pan for 10 minutes, then serve.

Store in an airtight container at room temperature for up to five days.

Cinnamon Oat Bites

Whether you're looking for a snack or a treat, these bites have just the right amount of sweetness to satisfy your yearnings. The flaxseeds and almond butter offer a nice balance of protein and healthy fats to curb cravings while supplying you with nutrients such as vitamin E and magnesium.

MAKES 16 BALLS | SERVES 6 TO 8 | PREP TIME: 15 MINUTES

- 3 pitted Medjool dates
- ½ cup unsweetened almond butter
- 1 tablespoon raw honey
- ¼ cup ground flaxseed
- ½ teaspoon ground cinnamon
- ½ teaspoon ground ginger
- 1 cup gluten-free rolled oats
- 2 to 4 tablespoons hot water
- 2 tablespoons raisins

In the bowl of a food processor fitted with the blade attachment, add the dates, almond butter, honey, flaxseed, cinnamon, and ginger, then pulse until chopped.

Add the oats and pulse until combined and a dough-like consistency forms. If needed, add 2 to 4 tablespoons of hot water to help the mixture come together. Add the raisins and pulse a couple of times just to incorporate them into the dough.

Roll the date mixture into 1-inch balls. Place the balls in an airtight container and store in the fridge for one week or in the freezer for one to two months.

Chocolate Truffles

Chocolate is known for its antioxidant properties, so here's your fall indulgence without processed sugar. Sweetened with dates and honey and balanced with nuts, seeds, and coconut oil, these truffles are the perfect energizing treat.

14 TRUFFLES | SERVES 6 TO 8 | PREP TIME: 20 MINUTES, PLUS 1 TO 2 HOURS FOR CHILLING

- ½ cup raw almonds
- ¼ cup pine nuts
- ¼ cup pumpkin seeds
- 5 pitted Medjool dates
- ⅛ teaspoon fine sea salt
- ½ teaspoon cinnamon

- ¼ cup unsweetened cocoa powder
- 2 tablespoons melted coconut oil
- 2 tablespoons melted raw honey
- Optional toppings: ½ cup unsweetened shredded coconut or ¼ cup goji berries

In the bowl of a food processor fitted with the blade attachment, add the almonds, pine nuts, pumpkin seeds, and dates. Once finely chopped, add salt, cinnamon, and cocoa powder, and blend for another minute. Add the melted coconut oil and honey, and pulse until a smooth dough forms. Form the dough into bite-size balls.

If desired, roll the balls in shredded coconut or top with a goji berry. Place on a plate lined with parchment or wax paper. Refrigerate for 1 to 2 hours before serving.

Store in an airtight container in the fridge for up to two weeks or in the freezer for up to two months.

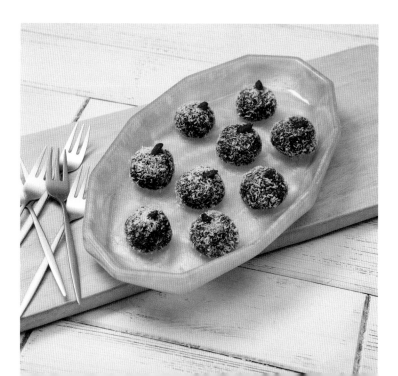

Pumpkin Pie with Almond Crust

It wouldn't be fall without pumpkin pie! This recipe is the ultimate in both flavor and tradition with a nutritional boost of antioxidants. The pumpkin filling is sweetened with dates and raw honey, and the coconut milk gives it a creamy texture on top of the almond crust.

ONE 9-INCH PIE | SERVES 6 TO 8 | PREP TIME: 20 MINUTES, PLUS SOAKING OVERNIGHT AND CHILLING FOR AT LEAST 2 HOURS | COOK TIME: 1 HOUR

ALMOND CRUST:
- 1 cup raw almonds
- 1 cup pitted Medjool dates
- 1 tablespoon melted coconut oil

PUMPKIN PIE FILLING:
- ½ cup pitted Medjool dates
- 1 cup pumpkin purée
- 2 tablespoons raw honey

- 1 (13.5-ounce) can unsweetened coconut cream
- 1 teaspoon vanilla extract
- 1½ teaspoons ground cinnamon
- 1½ teaspoons ground ginger
- ½ teaspoon ground nutmeg
- ⅛ teaspoon ground cloves
- ¼ teaspoon fine sea salt

FOR THE CRUST:

Place the almonds and dates in a bowl and cover with room-temperature water for at least 1 hour or as long as overnight.

Once soaked, drain the dates, and add them to the bowl of a food processor fitted with the blade attachment. Pulse until finely ground and the mixture resembles a paste.

Grease a 9-inch pie plate with coconut oil. Evenly press the date crust mixture into the bottom and sides of the pie plate. Chill in the refrigerator for at least 1 hour.

FOR THE FILLING:

Place the dates in a small bowl and cover with room-temperature water. Soak for at least 1 hour or as long as overnight.

Preheat the oven to 350°F.

Drain the dates and add them to the bowl of a food processor. Add the pumpkin purée, honey, coconut cream, vanilla, cinnamon, ginger, nutmeg, cloves, and salt. Pulse until very smooth and combined.

Pour the mixture onto the pie crust and smooth the top. Bake for 1 hour or until the filling is almost set and just slightly jiggles in the center (there will be cracks in the pie filling).

Remove the pie from the oven and allow to cool to room temperature. Then place in the refrigerator to fully set for at least 2 hours before serving.

Store the pie in the refrigerator for up to five days.

Kale Chips

Crunchy and salty are the keywords that make this the perfect snack. Add some spice to kick up the heat and arouse your taste buds. Replace potato chips with these fiber-, beta carotene-, and potassium-rich gems.

2 CUPS | SERVES 2 TO 4 | PREP TIME: 10 MINUTES | COOK TIME: 15 MINUTES

- 4 cups destemmed curly kale that has been torn into 2-inch pieces
- 1 tablespoon melted coconut oil
- ½ teaspoon garlic salt
- ½ teaspoon chili powder
- ½ teaspoon paprika
- 1 tablespoon nutritional yeast

Preheat the oven to 350°F.

Place the kale in a large bowl. Drizzle with coconut oil and sprinkle with garlic salt, chili powder, paprika, and nutritional yeast.

Toss the leaves in the oil and spices until evenly coated. Spread the kale on a baking sheet in a single layer.

Bake for 10 to 15 minutes, flipping halfway through, until crispy and lightly browned on the edges.

Remove the baking sheet from the oven and allow to cool on the baking sheet. The chips become crispier as they cool.

WINTER RECIPES

Barley Porridge with Pears

This warming and comforting barley breakfast is the perfect start to a winter day to help fight off the chill with some cinnamon and ginger. The maple syrup gives a nice sweetness along with the pear, while the high fiber from the barley and protein from the walnuts balance out the carbs. For a gluten-free version, substitute oats or buckwheat for the barley.

SERVES 2 | PREP TIME: 10 MINUTES | COOK TIME: 40 MINUTES

- 1 cup whole barley
- 3 cups water
- ¼ teaspoon sea salt
- 2 tablespoons maple syrup
- ½ cup unsweetened plain cashew milk
- ¼ teaspoon ground cinnamon
- ¼ teaspoon ground ginger or 1-inch piece fresh ginger, grated
- ½ cup diced pear
- ¼ cup chopped walnuts

Soak the barley in water for at least 1 hour. Drain the soaking water and rinse the barley. Add barley, water, and salt to a saucepan and bring to a boil. Reduce the heat and cook partially covered over medium heat for 30 to 40 minutes or until the barley is soft.

Remove the saucepan from the heat and add the maple syrup, cashew milk, cinnamon, ginger, pear, and walnuts. Serve warm.

Cinnamon Granola

Deliciously paired with a smoothie bowl or enjoyed on its own with some coconut or almond milk, this granola has winter's warm spice flavors and a tasty crunch.

SERVES 4 TO 5 | PREP TIME: 10 MINUTES | COOK TIME: 22 MINUTES

- 1 cup gluten-free rolled oats
- ½ cup chopped raw walnuts
- ½ cup unsweetened coconut chips or flakes
- ¼ cup raw sunflower seeds
- ¼ cup melted coconut oil

- ⅛ to ¼ cup maple syrup
- 1 teaspoon ground cinnamon
- 1 teaspoon vanilla extract
- ½ teaspoon sea salt

Preheat the oven to 325°F. Line a baking sheet with parchment paper.

Combine the oats, walnuts, coconut chips, and sunflower seeds in a medium bowl.

In a small bowl, mix together the coconut oil, maple syrup, cinnamon, vanilla, and salt. Drizzle over the oat mixture and toss to evenly coat.

Spread the mixture onto the prepared baking sheet. Bake for 20 to 22 minutes, stirring halfway through, until golden brown and fragrant. Allow to cool completely on the baking sheet. The granola will crisp as it cools.

Store in an airtight container at room temperature for up to one week.

Persimmon Smoothie Bowl

With a thick and velvety texture, this winter smoothie bowl is satisfying and nourishing. Since persimmons are high in vitamins A and C and the flaxseeds add some extra fiber, you're sure to start your morning right, especially when the smoothie bowl is topped with cinnamon granola!

SERVES 1 TO 2 | PREP TIME: 5 MINUTES

- 1 pitted Medjool date
- ¼ cup raw cashews or sunflower seeds
- 2 soft persimmons
- ¼ cup unsweetened plain cashew milk
- ½ cup diced ripe pear

- 1 tablespoon ground flaxseed
- ¼ teaspoon ground turmeric or fresh-peeled and grated turmeric
- ½ teaspoon vanilla extract

Place the date and cashews into a small bowl and cover with hot water. Allow to soak for 10 minutes to soften, then drain.

In the carafe of a high-speed blender, add the softened date and cashews, persimmons, cashew milk, pear, flaxseed, turmeric, and vanilla. Blend until smooth (the mixture will be very thick). Pour the mixture into a bowl and top with Cinnamon Granola (see recipe) or seasonal nuts.

Beet Ginger Smoothie Juice

You can enjoy this as a breakfast smoothie or a beverage on its own. Beets are full of nutrients such as folate and magnesium, and the celery, kale, apple, and hemp seeds give it an extra fiber punch.

SERVES 1 | PREP TIME: 5 MINUTES

- 1 small beet (4 ounces), peeled, scrubbed, and quartered (or grated if you don't have a high-powered blender)
- 1 small apple (5 ounces), cored and chopped
- 1 rib celery, chopped
- ½ cup kale
- 1 cup unsweetened plain cashew milk or filtered water
- 1 (1-inch piece) fresh ginger, peeled
- 1 tablespoon hemp seeds
- 1 lemon, juiced

In the carafe of a high-speed blender, add the beet, apple, celery, kale, cashew milk, ginger, hemp seeds, and lemon juice. Blend until smooth, and chill if desired before serving.

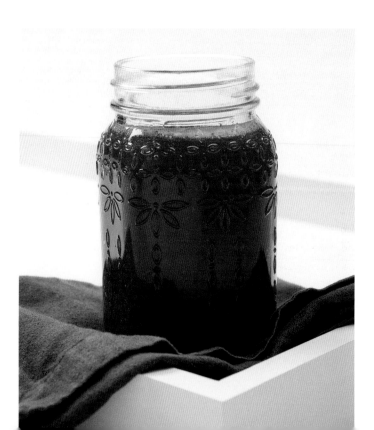

Warming Venison Stew

This comforting stew with meat and veggies cooked until tender helps warm us on a cool winter day. If you can't find venison locally, you can substitute with grass-fed beef or buffalo. The herbs and spices plus onion, carrots, and celery add extra antioxidant nourishment.

SERVES 4 TO 6 | PREP TIME: 15 MINUTES | COOK TIME: 1 HOUR

- 1 tablespoon avocado oil
- 1 pound venison stew meat
- 1 medium yellow onion, diced
- 4 medium carrots, peeled and thinly sliced (about 3 cups)
- 6 stalks celery, chopped (about 2 cups)
- 2 cloves garlic, peeled and crushed
- 2 bay leaves
- 1 teaspoon sea salt
- ½ teaspoon freshly ground black pepper
- ¼ teaspoon turmeric
- ⅛ teaspoon cayenne
- ⅛ teaspoon sweet paprika
- 2 teaspoons dried thyme
- 5 cups grass-fed beef or vegetable broth
- 1 (6-ounce) turnip or Yukon Gold potato, peeled and cut into 1-inch pieces (about 2 cups)

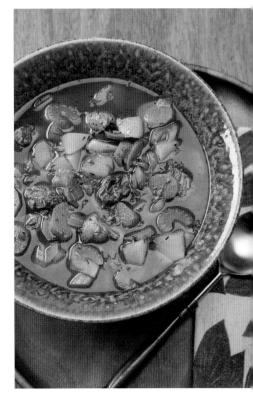

Heat the avocado oil in a large pot over medium heat. Add the venison and cook until browned on all sides but not cooked through, 6 to 8 minutes. Move the venison to a plate.

Add the onion, carrots, celery, and garlic, and cook until the onion is translucent and the vegetables have softened, 6 to 8 minutes. Add the bay leaves, salt, pepper, turmeric, cayenne, paprika, and thyme, and cook another minute or so until toasted and fragrant.

Deglaze the bottom of the pot with broth and add the turnip and venison. Bring to a boil, then reduce to a simmer. Allow to simmer for 45 minutes partially covered, adding water as necessary until the vegetables are tender and the meat is cooked through.

Remove and discard the bay leaves. Season to taste with salt and pepper again and serve warm.

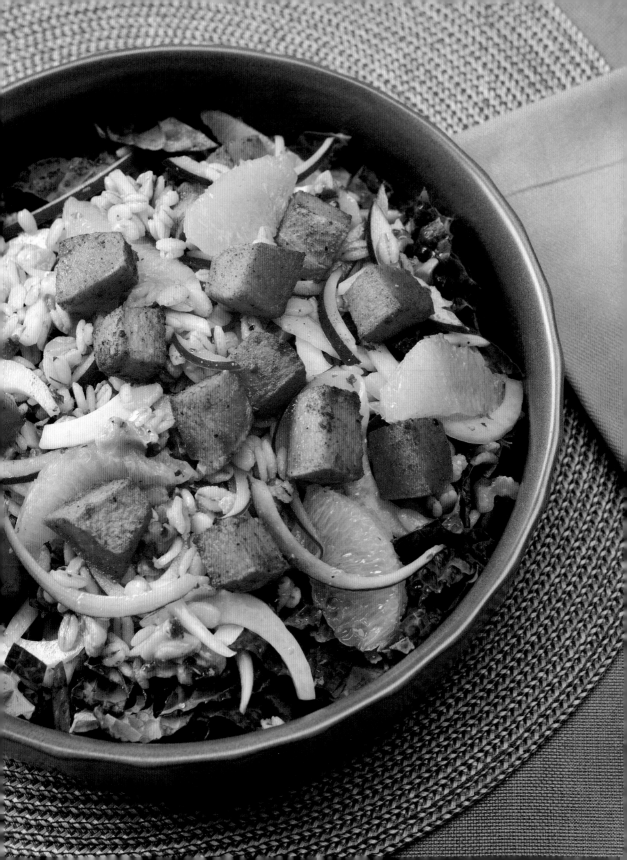

Barley Salad with Roasted Winter Squash

This flavorful, hearty salad is a classic seasonal combination of winter squash, fennel, onion, and orange. Together, these ingredients provide an array of immune-boosting nutrients, including vitamin C, beta carotene, selenium, and zinc. For a gluten-free version, substitute buckwheat for the barley.

SERVES 4 TO 6 | PREP TIME: 15 MINUTES | COOK TIME: 45 MINUTES

BARLEY SALAD:
- ⅔ cup whole barley, cooked according to package instructions (3 cups when cooked)
- 1 fennel bulb, thinly sliced
- ½ small red onion, thinly sliced
- ¼ cup chopped walnuts
- 1 cup destemmed and chopped lacinato kale
- 1 small orange, peeled and sliced

WINTER SQUASH:
- 2¼ pounds winter squash (butternut, acorn, buttercup, or delicata), peeled and cut into 1-inch cubes (5 cups)
- 1 tablespoon avocado oil

- 1 teaspoon ground ginger
- 1 teaspoon ground cinnamon
- ¼ teaspoon ground cloves
- 1 tablespoon maple syrup
- Sea salt and freshly ground black pepper to taste

DRESSING:
- ¼ cup extra-virgin olive oil
- 2 tablespoons apple cider vinegar
- 1 teaspoon dried oregano
- 1 teaspoon Dijon mustard
- 1 teaspoon maple syrup
- Sea salt and freshly ground black pepper to taste

FOR THE BARLEY SALAD:

In a large bowl, add the barley, fennel bulb, red onion, walnuts, kale, and orange.

FOR THE ROASTED WINTER SQUASH:

Preheat the oven to 400°F. Line a baking sheet with parchment paper.

Combine the squash, avocado oil, ginger, cinnamon, cloves, maple syrup, and salt and pepper, and toss to evenly coat. Roast, flipping halfway through, until golden brown and tender, 30 to 35 minutes.

FOR THE DRESSING:

Whisk together the olive oil, vinegar, oregano, mustard, and maple syrup. Drizzle the dressing around the rim of the salad bowl and toss to evenly coat the salad. Season with salt and pepper as desired and top with the roasted winter squash.

Baked Quail with Roasted Parsnips

This savory winter roast has tender veggies and apple for a flavorful and nourishing boost. If you can't find quail locally, you can use free-range chicken thighs instead and increase the roast time to 30 to 35 minutes or until 165°F on the thermometer.

SERVES 4 | PREP TIME: 15 MINUTES | COOK TIME: 20 MINUTES

- 4 (4 to 5 ounces) whole quail, cleaned and rinsed
- 2 tablespoons avocado oil
- ½ teaspoon sea salt
- ¼ teaspoon ground pepper
- 1 carrot, diced
- 1 celery stalk, diced
- 2 large parsnips, peeled and cubed
- 2 shallots, peeled and diced
- 1 organic apple, unpeeled, cored, and sliced
- ½ teaspoon ground turmeric
- 1 teaspoon blend of dried thyme, basil, rosemary, and sage
- ½ teaspoon sea salt
- ¼ teaspoon ground pepper
- ⅓ cup apple juice or broth
- ¼ cup parsley, chopped for garnish

Preheat the oven to 450°F.

Rinse the quail and place them in a large baking dish.

Coat the quail with avocado oil, salt, and pepper. Add the carrot, celery, parsnips, shallots, and apple to the baking dish. Sprinkle with turmeric, dried herbs, salt, and pepper, and pour in the apple juice. Bake for 15 to 20 minutes or until the meat is slightly firm, the juices run clear, and the temperature on a meat thermometer registers 165°F. Garnish with chopped parsley and serve warm.

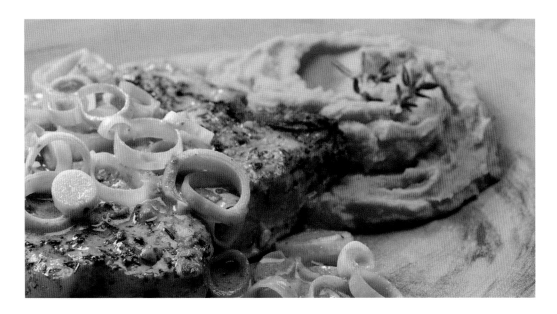

Pork Chops with Leeks and Mashed Yams

I grew up in the South, and pork chops and yams were a staple meal in the winters. My mother grew up on a pig farm, and we always had neighbors who raised hogs. This simple and savory pork chop recipe is topped with tender flavonoid-rich leeks and paired with sweet potatoes with a touch of winter spices.

SERVES 4 | PREP TIME: 20 MINUTES | COOK TIME: 35 MINUTES

PORK CHOPS:
- 4 pasture-raised bone-in pork chops, 1½ inches thick (about 2¾ pounds)
- 1 tablespoon avocado oil
- ¼ teaspoon sea salt
- ¼ teaspoon freshly ground black pepper
- ½ teaspoon dried thyme
- ½ teaspoon dried basil
- ½ teaspoon dried rosemary
- 3 leeks, white and light green parts only, thinly sliced
- ½ cup diced yellow onion
- ⅓ cup chicken broth
- 2 tablespoons Dijon mustard
- 3 cloves garlic, minced

MASHED YAMS:
- 2 large yams (about 1 pound, 10 ounces), peeled and cut into 1-inch-thick
- ½ teaspoon ground ginger or fresh ginger, peeled and grated
- ½ teaspoon ground cinnamon
- ¼ teaspoon ground nutmeg
- ¼ cup unsweetened plain nut milk
- 2 tablespoons coconut oil or ghee
- ½ teaspoon sea salt
- 2 teaspoons maple syrup

FOR THE PORK CHOPS:

Preheat the oven to 350°F.

Coat the pork chops with avocado oil and place them in a baking dish. Sprinkle with salt, pepper, thyme, basil, and rosemary. Top with the leeks and onion. Whisk the broth, mustard, and garlic together in a measuring cup and pour over everything.

Bake for 30 to 35 minutes or until the chops reach an internal temperature of 145°F.

FOR THE MASHED YAMS:

Place a steamer basket in a large pot and fill with 1 inch of water. Bring to a simmer. Add the yams and cover the pot with a lid. Allow to steam for 15 to 20 minutes until very tender when pierced with a knife.

Remove the yams carefully to the bowl of a food processor fitted with the blade attachment. Add the ginger, cinnamon, nutmeg, nut milk, coconut oil, salt, and maple syrup. Serve with the pork chops.

Bison Meatloaf with Garlic Broccoli

The garlic and sun-dried tomatoes give this meatloaf a nice flavor, and it's the perfect warm comfort food for winter. Bison is rich in iron, selenium, and zinc, which are important nutrients for winter months.

SERVES 2 TO 3 | PREP TIME: 10 MINUTES | COOK TIME: 30 MINUTES

BISON MEATLOAF:

- Avocado or coconut oil spray, for greasing
- 1 pound ground bison meat
- 1 large egg
- ½ cup gluten-free breadcrumbs or gluten-free rolled oats
- 2 tablespoons chopped sun-dried tomatoes
- 1 teaspoon sea salt
- ½ teaspoon freshly ground black pepper
- ½ small yellow onion, grated on the large holes of a box grater
- 1 medium carrot, peeled and grated on the large holes of a box grater
- 1 tablespoon Italian seasoning or a combination of oregano, rosemary, marjoram, and thyme

GARLIC BROCCOLI:

- 1 tablespoon avocado oil
- 5 cloves minced garlic
- 14 ounces (about 5 cups) broccoli florets, cut into ½-inch pieces
- ½ teaspoon sea salt
- ¼ cup spring or filtered water

FOR THE BISON MEATLOAF:

Preheat the oven to 350°F. Grease a 9 × 5–inch loaf pan with cooking spray.

Combine the bison, egg, breadcrumbs, sun-dried tomatoes, salt, pepper, onion, carrot, and Italian seasoning. Mix with your hands if necessary.

Press into the loaf pan evenly and bake for 30 minutes or until a meat thermometer registers 160°F. Allow to cool for 10 minutes in the loaf pan, then remove. Slice and serve with garlic broccoli.

FOR THE GARLIC BROCCOLI:

Heat the avocado oil in a large sauté pan over medium heat. Add garlic and cook, stirring frequently, for 1 to 2 minutes, but do not burn the garlic. Add broccoli, salt, and water. Cover and steam until crisp-tender but not overcooked, 4 to 5 minutes. Serve immediately with bison meatloaf.

Black Bean and Swiss Chard Soup

Warming cayenne and paprika give this soup extra heat to keep you toasty through wintertime. The high fiber and antioxidant content help support hormonal harmony.

SERVES 4 TO 6 | PREP TIME: 15 MINUTES | COOK TIME: 35 MINUTES

- 1 tablespoon avocado oil
- 1 small onion, diced
- 2 cloves garlic, minced
- 4 cups vegetable or free-range chicken broth
- 1 tablespoon dried parsley
- 1 tablespoon dried oregano
- ¼ teaspoon cayenne
- 1 teaspoon paprika
- ½ teaspoon sea salt
- 15-ounce can or 2 cups cooked black beans, drained and rinsed
- 3 cups chopped Swiss chard
- Freshly ground black pepper to taste

Heat the avocado oil in a large pot over medium heat. Sauté the onion and garlic until the onion is translucent, about 4 minutes. Add the broth, parsley, oregano, cayenne, paprika, salt, and beans, and bring the soup to a boil.

Reduce the heat to medium-low and simmer for 15 minutes. Stir in the chard and continue simmering for 10 to 15 minutes. Season with salt and pepper as needed.

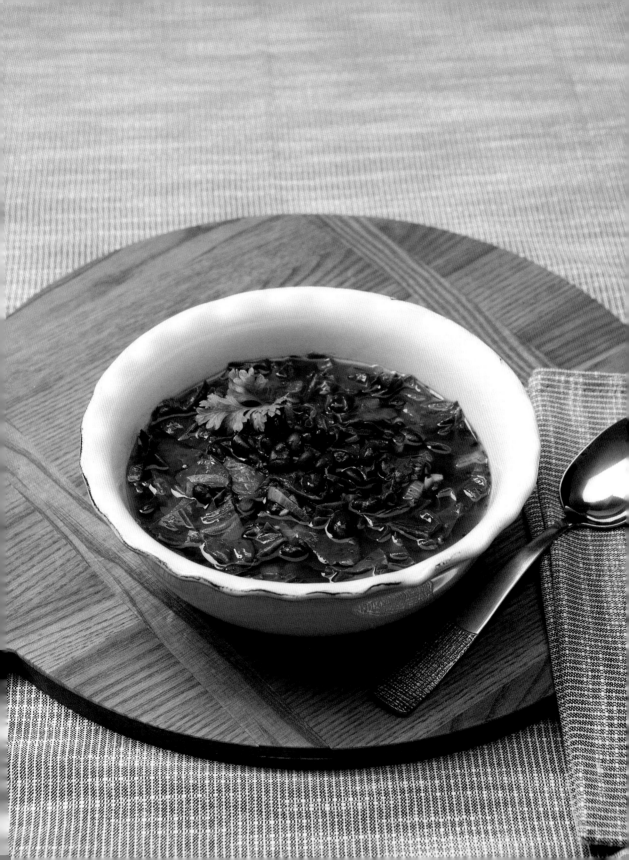

Winter Squash Soup

This clean squash soup, rich in beta carotene and B vitamins, warms your body, and topping it with pumpkin seeds adds a nice crunch.

SERVES 3 TO 5 | PREP TIME: 15 MINUTES | COOK TIME: 30 MINUTES

- 2 tablespoons coconut oil
- 1 white onion, diced
- 4 cloves garlic, sliced
- ½ teaspoon cinnamon
- ½ teaspoon cumin
- 1 teaspoon sea salt
- 2 cups peeled, cubed pumpkin (or other winter squash)
- 2 cups peeled, cubed butternut squash
- 3 cups chicken bone broth or veggie stock
- 1 tablespoon maple syrup
- ¼ cup pumpkin seeds

Heat the coconut oil in a large pot over medium heat. Add the onion and garlic and cook until softened, about 4 minutes.

Add the cinnamon, cumin, salt, pumpkin, and butternut squash, and cook another minute to toast the spices and coat the squash. Deglaze the pan with the bone broth and bring to a boil. Reduce to a simmer for 10 to 12 minutes or until the squash is tender. Stir in the maple syrup.

Working in batches, transfer the soup to the carafe of a blender and purée until smooth, adding more broth or water as necessary for consistency. Serve warm topped with pumpkin seeds.

Potato Leek Soup

Looking for a winter comfort food? This soup is creamy and deliciously comforting. Leeks and potatoes are gut nourishing without the dairy, which is a common digestive irritant.

SERVES 4 TO 5 | **PREP TIME: 15 MINUTES** | **COOK TIME: 40 MINUTES**

- 2 tablespoons avocado oil
- 3 large leeks, white and light green parts only, thinly sliced
- 1 medium yellow or white onion, chopped
- 4 cloves garlic, minced
- 1 teaspoon sea salt
- ¼ teaspoon ground pepper
- 1 teaspoon dried thyme or 2 teaspoons fresh thyme, plus more for garnish
- 1 teaspoon dried sage or 1½ teaspoons chopped fresh sage leaves
- 1 teaspoon dried rosemary or 1 teaspoon chopped fresh rosemary leaves
- 2 bay leaves
- 4 medium (2 pounds) Yukon Gold potatoes, peeled and chopped (about 5¼ cups)
- 5 cups vegetable broth
- 1 cup unsweetened cashew nut milk

Heat the avocado oil in a large heavy-bottomed pot over medium heat. Add the leeks, onion, and garlic, and sauté until soft, about 5 minutes. Add the salt, pepper, thyme, sage, rosemary, bay leaves, potatoes, and broth.

Bring to a boil, then reduce to a simmer. Allow to simmer for 20 minutes or until the potatoes are tender. Stir in the milk and season with additional salt and pepper to taste.

In batches, remove the mixture to the carafe of a blender and blend until smooth. Serve garnished with additional fresh thyme leaves if desired.

––––––––––––

Tip: Another fun topping for the omnivores out there is cooked chopped bacon.

Salmon Cabbage Salad

While fresh-caught wild salmon is hard to find in winter, you can still get the omega-3 fatty acid benefits from canned or frozen wild salmon. This recipe is full of flavor, and the cabbage gives the salmon salad a nice crunchy texture.

SERVES 4 | PREP TIME: 15 MINUTES

SALMON SALAD:
- 1 (15-ounce) can wild Alaskan salmon, drained
- 2 to 3 ribs celery, thinly sliced (about 1 cup)
- ½ cup diced red onion
- 1 tablespoon extra-virgin olive oil
- 1 tablespoon fresh lemon juice
- 2 teaspoons Dijon mustard
- 1 tablespoon dried dill or 2 tablespoons fresh dill
- ¼ cup chopped fresh parsley
- 1 teaspoon cumin
- ¼ teaspoon sea salt
- ⅛ teaspoon ground black pepper

CABBAGE:
- 8 cups shredded green cabbage
- 1 lemon, juiced
- 2 tablespoons extra-virgin olive oil
- ¼ teaspoon sea salt

FOR THE SALMON SALAD:

Combine the salmon, celery, red onion, olive oil, lemon juice, mustard, dill, parsley, cumin, salt, and pepper. Set aside.

FOR THE CABBAGE:

In a large bowl, add the cabbage and drizzle the lemon juice, olive oil, and salt around the rim of the bowl. Toss to coat well. Divide the cabbage among four plates and top with the salmon salad.

Endive Lentil Salad with Shallot Herb Dressing

Winter flavors abound in this salad filled with squash, lentils, endive, and apples with herbs to give the antioxidant level an extra lift.

SERVES 2 TO 3 | **PREP TIME: 15 MINUTES** | **COOK TIME: 22 MINUTES**

ENDIVE LENTIL SALAD:
- 2 cups peeled and cut butternut squash (1-inch cubes)
- 1 tablespoon avocado oil
- ¼ teaspoon sea salt
- ¼ teaspoon freshly ground pepper
- ⅓ cup green lentils, cooked according to package instructions
- 4 cups endive, thinly sliced
- 2 red apples, cored and diced (about 2½ cups)
- ¼ cup parsley leaves

SHALLOT HERB DRESSING:
- 1 lemon, juiced
- 3 tablespoons extra-virgin olive oil
- 1 tablespoon minced shallot
- ½ teaspoon dried thyme or 1 teaspoon fresh thyme leaves
- ½ teaspoon dried oregano or 1 teaspoon chopped fresh oregano leaves
- Salt to taste
- Pepper to taste
- 2 tablespoons pine nuts, toasted

FOR THE ENDIVE LENTIL SALAD:

Preheat the oven to 400°F.

Toss the butternut squash cubes with avocado oil, salt, and pepper, and bake for 18 to 22 minutes until golden and tender. Allow to cool slightly once finished.

Meanwhile, cook the lentils according to the package instructions until tender and rinse under cold water to stop the cooking. Set aside.

Combine the endive, apples, cooked lentils, parsley, and baked squash in a large bowl.

FOR THE SHALLOT HERB DRESSING:

In a small bowl, whisk together lemon juice, olive oil, shallot, thyme, and oregano. Season with salt and pepper to taste. Drizzle the dressing around the rim of the salad bowl and toss to evenly coat. Sprinkle with pine nuts and serve.

Tip: To toast the pine nuts, place the pine nuts in a small sauté pan over medium heat. Allow to toast until golden, fragrant, and nutty, 3 to 5 minutes. Remove to a small bowl to cool.

Nut Crackers with Black Bean Dip

Curled up reading a book or catching up with friends is the perfect time to munch on this delicious crunchy and nutty snack. With a garlic kick, you're sure to get your dose of immune-boosting allicin.

1½ CUPS DIP AND 20 CRACKERS | SERVES 6 TO 10 | PREP TIME: 10 MINUTES, PLUS 1 HOUR FOR FREEZING | COOK TIME: 35 MINUTES

NUT CRACKERS:
- 1 cup raw cashews
- 1 cup raw walnuts
- ¼ cup hemp seeds
- ¼ cup filtered water
- 3 tablespoons extra-virgin olive oil
- 1 teaspoon sea salt
- ¼ teaspoon garlic powder

BLACK BEAN DIP:
- 1 (15-ounce) can black beans, drained and rinsed, or 1½ cups cooked black beans
- 2 tablespoons extra-virgin olive oil
- ¼ cup tahini, well-stirred
- 1 lemon, juiced
- 1 clove garlic
- ½ teaspoon ground cumin
- Pinch chili powder
- Pinch cayenne pepper
- Pinch sweet paprika
- ½ teaspoon sea salt
- 5 tablespoons water

FOR THE NUT CRACKERS:

In a food processor fitted with the blade attachment, add the cashews, walnuts, and hemp seeds. Pulse the nuts and seeds until the texture is like coarse sand. Add the water and blend again. Then add the olive oil, salt, and garlic powder, and blend until a dough forms.

Move the dough to a piece of parchment paper and roll it to form a 2-inch-in-diameter log. Place in the freezer until firm enough to slice (about 1 hour).

Preheat the oven to 350°F. Line a baking sheet with parchment paper. With a serrated knife, slice the dough about ¼ to ½ inch thick.

Bake the crackers until their edges and bottoms are golden brown, 30 to 35 minutes. Let cool on the baking sheet and serve at room temperature.

FOR THE BLACK BEAN DIP:

In a food processor fitted with the blade attachment, combine the beans, olive oil, tahini, lemon juice, garlic, cumin, chili powder, cayenne pepper, paprika, salt, and water. Pulse until very smooth. Move to an airtight container and refrigerate until ready to use. Serve with the nut crackers. Store the dip in the refrigerator for up to three days.

Gluten-Free Gingerbread Muffins

Whether you're looking for a treat, snack, or breakfast on the go, these muffins with winter spices and molasses are sure to please your palate. If you use a premade gluten-free flour blend and it already contains xanthan gum, baking soda, and baking powder, skip those ingredients.

MAKES 12 MUFFINS | **SERVES 12** | **PREP TIME: 15 MINUTES** | **COOK TIME: 20 MINUTES**

- Avocado or coconut cooking spray
- 2 cups gluten-free flour (equal parts tapioca, coconut, and rice flours)
- ½ teaspoon xanthan gum
- ¼ teaspoon baking soda
- 1 teaspoon baking powder
- 1 teaspoon ground cinnamon
- 2 teaspoons ground ginger
- ¼ teaspoon ground cloves
- ¼ teaspoon ground nutmeg
- ½ teaspoon sea salt
- ½ cup unsweetened applesauce
- ¼ cup unsulfured molasses
- ½ cup maple syrup
- 6 tablespoons melted unsalted butter or coconut oil

Preheat the oven to 350°F. Grease a 12-cup muffin tin with cooking spray.

In a large bowl, whisk together the flour, xanthan gum, baking soda, baking powder, cinnamon, ginger, cloves, nutmeg, and salt.

In a separate medium bowl, whisk the applesauce, molasses, maple syrup, and butter until combined.

Make a well in the flour mixture, add the applesauce mixture into the center of the well, and then stir gently until a batter forms.

Divide the batter among the muffin molds, filling each mold three-quarters of the way full. Bake for 18 to 20 minutes or until an inserted toothpick comes out clean. Allow to cool in the pan for 10 minutes, then remove to cool further on a wire baking rack.

Store in an airtight container at room temperature for up to five days.

Baked Apples

These tender and sweet warm apples topped with oats and walnuts are a mouthwatering dessert to help bring a nourishing end to your winter day.

SERVES 4 | PREP TIME: 15 MINUTES | COOK TIME: 45 MINUTES

- 1 tablespoon melted coconut oil
- ¼ cup old-fashioned rolled oats
- 6 tablespoons chopped walnuts
- 2 teaspoons ground cinnamon
- ¼ teaspoon nutmeg
- 2 teaspoons pure vanilla extract
- 2 tablespoons maple syrup
- 4 organic, late-season apples, cored
- ½ cup apple juice

Preheat the oven to 350°F. Place the apples in a 8 × 8–inch baking dish.

Combine the coconut oil, oats, walnuts, cinnamon, nutmeg, vanilla, and maple syrup. Stuff the oat mixture into the center of each apple. Pour the apple juice into the bottom of the baking dish. Cover with foil and bake for 40 to 45 minutes or until the apples are very tender. Allow to cool for 15 minutes, then serve.

Carrot Salad

Indulge your taste buds with this crisp, fresh snack while providing your body with an energizing boost of antioxidants and nutty protein.

SERVES 4 | PREP TIME: 15 MINUTES, PLUS TIME FOR CHILLING

- 2 cups peeled and grated carrots (use the large holes of a box grater)
- ½ cup diced celery
- ¼ cup raisins
- 1 medium apple, cored and chopped
- ¼ cup chopped raw cashews
- 3 to 4 tablespoons cashew nut milk
- 1 tablespoon extra-virgin olive oil
- Pinch ground cumin
- 3 tablespoons chopped parsley
- Sea salt and freshly ground black pepper to taste

Combine the carrots, celery, raisins, apple, cashews, nut milk, olive oil, cumin, and parsley, and toss to combine. Season with salt and pepper to taste. Cover and chill in the refrigerator for several hours before serving.

SPRING RECIPES

Spring Greens Smoothie

Buzz into spring flavors and bump up your vitamin C with the natural sweetness of fresh strawberries and spring greens.

SERVES 1 | PREP TIME: 5 MINUTES

- 1 cup unsweetened cashew nut milk
- ¼ cup chopped cilantro, parsley, or mint
- ¼ cup raw cashews
- 1 cup spring greens
- 1 lemon, juiced
- ½ cup frozen or fresh strawberries

Add the cashew milk, cilantro, cashews, greens, lemon juice, and strawberries to the carafe of a blender, and blend until smooth. Chill in the refrigerator if desired, then pour into a glass to serve.

Kiwi Mint Smoothie with Bee Pollen

Start your spring morning with a tangy and crisp smoothie with a hint of sweetness. Add some bee pollen to help balance your immune system so you can sail through allergy season with ease.

SERVES 1 | PREP TIME: 5 MINUTES

- 1 ripe kiwi, peeled
- 6 mint leaves
- 1 cup lettuce greens
- 1 cup unsweetened macadamia nut milk
- ½ lemon, juiced
- 2 teaspoons raw honey or maple syrup
- 1 tablespoon bee pollen (granules or powder)

Combine the kiwi, mint, lettuce greens, milk, lemon juice, honey, and bee pollen in the carafe of a blender and blend until smooth. Chill until ready to serve. Serve in a tall glass.

Poached Eggs over Arugula and Sprouts Bowl

Spring chickens are laying fresh eggs so it's the time for poached eggs paired with fresh seasonal greens for a B vitamin boost.

SERVES 2 | PREP TIME: 15 MINUTES | COOK TIME: 5 MINUTES

- 1 tablespoon apple cider vinegar
- 4 large eggs
- 1 cup dandelion greens (or other seasonal spring greens)
- 2 cups arugula
- 1 cup green-leaf sprouts (such as broccoli sprouts) or microgreens
- ½ cup thinly sliced radishes
- 3 tablespoons extra-virgin olive oil
- 1 lemon, juiced
- 2 tablespoons chopped spring onions
- Sea salt and freshly ground black pepper to taste

Fill a large deep skillet three-quarters full with water, add the vinegar, and bring to a slow simmer over medium-low heat.

When the water is at a slow simmer, make a circular motion using a large, slotted spoon to create a whirlpool effect. Break an egg into a cup and then gently slip the egg into the simmering water. Allow the egg to swirl and begin to cook. Continue cooking for 3 to 5 minutes until the white is cooked through but the yolk is still runny. Remove to a cool bowl of a water and repeat with the remaining eggs. Set aside.

Meanwhile, place the greens, arugula, sprouts, and radishes in a large bowl. Whisk together the olive oil, lemon juice, and salt and pepper to taste in a small bowl. Drizzle the dressing around the rim of the large bowl with the greens and toss them to evenly combine and coat in the dressing. Divide the greens between two plates, top with spring onions and poached eggs, and season with additional salt and pepper.

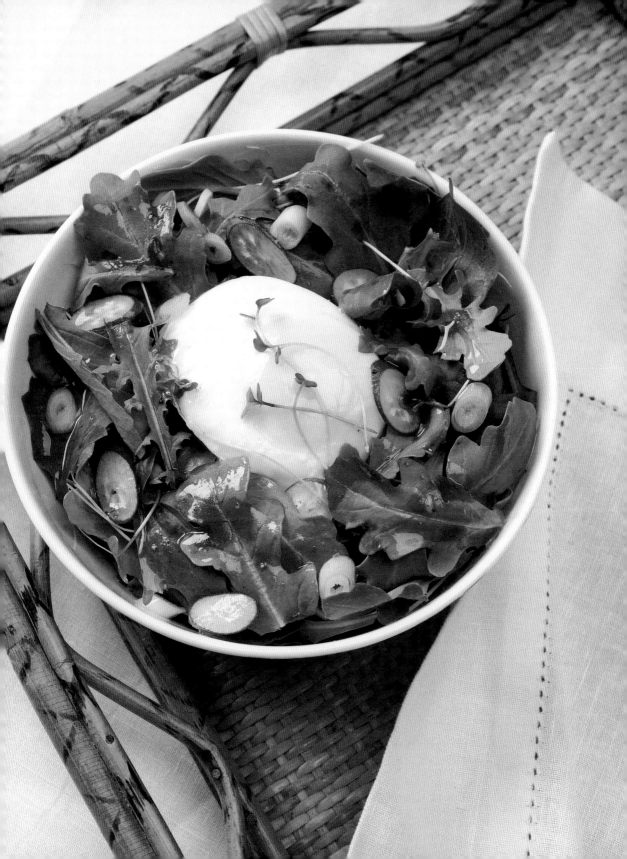

Dandelion Strawberry Bowl with Macadamia Nuts

Spring into your day with a dandelion strawberry smoothie bowl packed full of fresh flavors and hormone-balancing nourishment and topped with a macadamia crunch.

SERVES 1 | PREP TIME: 5 MINUTES

- 1 cup dandelion greens
- 1 cup macadamia nut milk
- ½ cup frozen or fresh strawberries
- 1 ripe apricot, pit removed (optional, if available)
- 1 cup green-leaf sprouts or microgreens, divided
- ¼ cup chopped macadamia nuts, divided
- ½ to 1 teaspoon maple syrup (optional)

Combine the dandelion greens, nut milk, strawberries, apricot, ½ cup sprouts, 2 tablespoons macadamia nuts, and maple syrup. Blend until smooth, periodically mixing with a spatula (this mixture will be very thick).

Pour the mixture into a bowl and top with the remaining macadamia nuts and sprouts. If more sweetness is desired, drizzle with maple syrup.

LUNCH AND DINNER

Pan Seared Scallops over Collard Greens

Fresh scallops are easier to find in springtime and what better way to enjoy them than over a bed of newly harvested collard greens.

SERVES 2 TO 3 | PREP TIME: 15 MINUTES | COOK TIME: 10 MINUTES

COLLARD GREENS:
- 3 cups chopped collard greens
- 1 to 2 tablespoon extra-virgin olive oil
- Sea salt to taste

PAN SEARED SCALLOPS:
- 3 tablespoons avocado oil
- 1 pound raw scallops (fresh or frozen)

- ½ teaspoon sea salt
- Freshly ground black pepper to taste
- 5 green (spring) garlic stalks, slice the white and light green leaves and the first few inches of the dark-green leaves, or 3 garlic cloves, crushed
- 2 tablespoons lemon juice
- 2 tablespoons chopped fresh parsley
- 2 tablespoons chopped fresh chives

FOR THE COLLARD GREENS:

In a large bowl, drizzle the collard greens with olive oil and season with sea salt. Using your hands, massage the collard greens with the oil and salt until they are slightly wilted and tender. Set aside until ready to serve.

FOR THE SCALLOPS:

If the scallops are frozen, thaw them in cold water. Heat the avocado oil in a large heavy-bottomed skillet over medium-high heat. Pat the scallops very dry and season with salt and pepper.

Place in the skillet and cook for about 2 to 3 minutes on each side until golden brown and opaque. Remove from the heat and garnish with the garlic, lemon juice, parsley, and chives.

Serve warm over the collard greens.

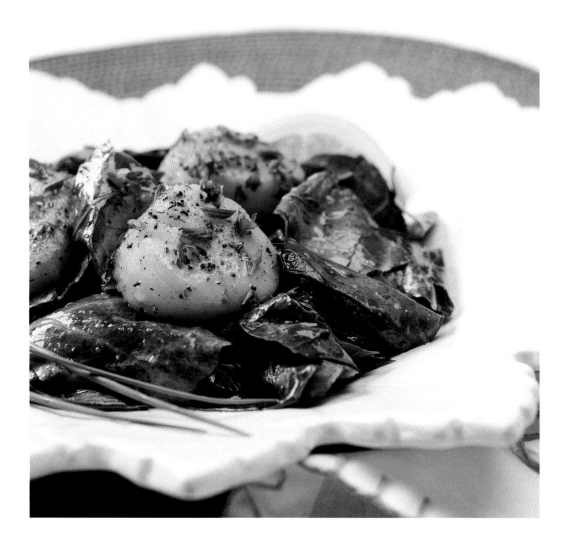

Spring Chive Soup

This soup is ideal for that cooler spring day when the sun hasn't quite warmed your body. It's comforting and rich in flavor with green onions and chives and creaminess from nut milk.

SERVES 2 | PREP TIME: 15 MINUTES | COOK TIME: 25 MINUTES

- 1 tablespoon avocado oil
- 4 green garlic stalks or 2 cloves garlic
- ¼ cup thinly sliced green onions
- 2 tablespoons gluten-free all-purpose flour
- 2 cups vegetable broth
- 3 cups chopped new potatoes (1 pound)

- 1 cup unsweetened cashew nut milk
- 1 tablespoon ghee or grass-fed butter (optional)
- ½ teaspoon sea salt
- ¼ teaspoon black pepper
- ¼ cup thinly sliced fresh chives

Heat the oil in a medium saucepan over medium-high heat. Add the garlic and green onions and cook until softened, about 1 minute. Whisk the flour into the pan and cook for another minute.

Add the broth, potatoes, cashew milk, ghee, salt, and pepper to the pan, and bring to a boil. Cover, reduce heat to low, and allow to simmer for about 15 minutes or until the potatoes are tender. Remove the pan from the heat and mash the potato mixture with a potato masher to a smooth consistency.

Divide among two bowls and garnish with 1 to 2 teaspoons of sliced chives.

Pacific Sardines Salad

Pacific sardines are more abundant in spring, and adding them to a salad with microgreens, parsley, and radishes is a fitting combination for drifting into warmer days.

SERVES 3 TO 4 | PREP TIME: 15 MINUTES

- 2 (3.75-ounce) cans pacific sardines, drained
- 2 tablespoons extra-virgin olive oil
- 1 tablespoon lemon juice
- 1 tablespoon avocado mayonnaise
- ½ tablespoon Dijon mustard
- 2 tablespoons chopped fresh parsley

- ½ cup minced radishes
- ¼ cup chopped spring onions or scallions
- Sea salt and freshly ground black pepper to taste
- 4 cups spring greens
- 1 cup green-leaf sprouts or microgreens

Mash the sardines in a medium bowl using a fork. Add the oil, lemon juice, mayonnaise, mustard, parsley, radishes, and onions. Season with salt and pepper, and mix to combine. Serve the sardine salad over the spring greens and top with the sprouts.

Creamy Cilantro Green Pea Soup

The vibrant green color and crisp flavors of this creamy pea soup has cilantro, which adds extra vitamin C to energize your body for spring.

SERVES 2 | PREP TIME: 15 MINUTES | COOK TIME: 25 MINUTES

- 2 tablespoons avocado oil
- ¼ cup chopped green onions
- 4 cups vegetable stock
- 4 cups frozen or fresh green peas
- 1 cup peeled and diced new potatoes
- ½ cup unsweetened cashew milk
- ½ teaspoon sea salt
- ½ cup cilantro
- Pinch freshly ground black pepper

In a large pot over medium heat, heat the oil and sauté the green onions until soft, a minute or so. Add the vegetable stock, peas, potatoes, cashew milk, and salt, and bring to a boil.

Reduce the heat to low, cover, and simmer for 10 to 15 minutes or until the potatoes and peas are soft. Remove from the heat and add the cilantro and pepper. Working in batches, transfer the soup into the carafe of a blender and process the mixture until smooth. Serve warm or cold.

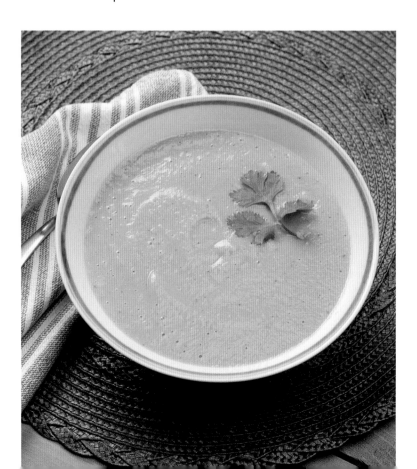

Asparagus and Fava Bean Salad

Classic spring flavors abound in this salad with crisp-tender veggies. Rich favas, lemon, and fresh herbs brighten all the ingredients.

SERVES 4 TO 6 | PREP TIME: 20 MINUTES | COOK TIME: 5 MINUTES

ASPARAGUS AND FAVA BEAN SALAD:
- 2 cups shelled fava beans (about 3 pounds)
- 1 (1-pound) bunch asparagus, trimmed

DRESSING:
- ½ lemon, zested
- 1 tablespoon fresh lemon juice
- 2 tablespoons apple cider vinegar
- ¼ cup extra-virgin olive oil
- ½ teaspoon sea salt
- 2 tablespoons chopped fresh mint
- 2 tablespoons chopped fresh parsley
- 2 tablespoons chopped chives

FOR THE SALAD:

Fill a medium saucepan with salted water and heat to a boil. Set up an ice bath next to the stove. Blanch the fava beans in the water for about a minute, then use a slotted spoon to move them to the ice water to stop the cooking.

Once the fava beans have cooled, use the slotted spoon to remove them from the ice water. Peel and discard the outer skin of the beans. Place the peeled favas into a medium bowl.

Place the asparagus into the boiling water and blanch for 3 to 4 minutes until the asparagus is bright green and crisp-tender. Move the asparagus to the ice water with the slotted spoon. Then add the asparagus to the bowl with the fava beans, using the slotted spoon again. Set aside.

FOR THE DRESSING:

In a separate small bowl, whisk together the lemon zest, lemon juice, vinegar, oil, and salt. Add the mint, parsley, and chives, and stir to combine.

Toss the dressing with the favas and asparagus, and serve at room temperature or chill in the refrigerator in an airtight container prior to serving.

Spring Greens and Strawberry Salad

Salads are precisely the nourishment our bodies need to shift from winter to spring, with easy-to-digest, tender, early warm-weather greens, mint, scallions, and light dressings like ones in this recipe.

SERVES 3 TO 4 | PREP TIME: 15 MINUTES

DRESSING:
- 3 tablespoons extra-virgin olive oil
- 2 tablespoons balsamic vinegar
- 1 teaspoon Dijon mustard
- 1 teaspoon pure maple syrup
- ¼ teaspoon sea salt
- Pinch freshly ground black pepper
- 2 tablespoons chopped mint

SPRING GREENS AND
STRAWBERRY SALAD:
- 6 cups mix of spring greens
- 2 cups quartered strawberries
- ¼ cup thinly sliced scallions
- 1 cup chopped macadamia nuts

FOR THE DRESSING:
Whisk together the oil, vinegar, mustard, maple syrup, salt, pepper, and mint in a small bowl.

FOR THE SALAD:
In a large salad bowl, mix the spring greens, strawberries, scallions, and nuts. Drizzle the dressing around the rim of the bowl and toss to evenly coat everything. Serve.

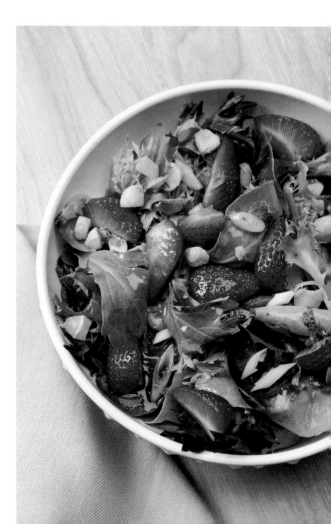

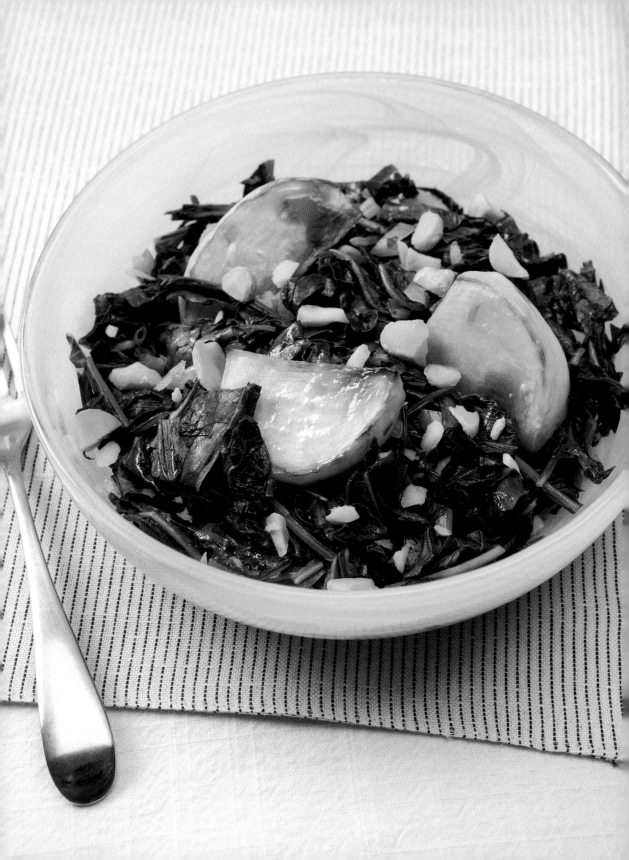

Braised Turnips and Greens Bowl

As the ground starts to warm up in spring, it's time to harvest turnips before we shift into the hot days of summer. This recipe pairs them with warm mustard greens and broth, making this the perfect early spring seasonal dish.

SERVES 2 TO 3 | PREP TIME: 10 MINUTES | COOK TIME: 15 MINUTES

- 5 medium turnips
- 2 tablespoons avocado oil
- 2 green garlic stalks or green onions, minced
- 1 cup vegetable broth
- 1 tablespoon lemon juice
- ⅛ teaspoon sea salt
- ¼ teaspoon ground black pepper
- 1 cup mustard greens
- 1 teaspoon maple syrup
- ½ cup chopped raw macadamia nuts

Trim, peel, and quarter the turnips, and then chop the turnip greens.

Heat the avocado oil in a medium saucepan over medium heat. Add the turnips and garlic, and cook for 5 minutes or until the turnips are golden on each side.

Add the broth, lemon juice, salt, and pepper, and bring to a boil. Cover and reduce the heat to a simmer. Allow to simmer until the turnips are slightly tender, about 5 to 10 minutes.

Increase the temperature to medium-high heat, add the greens, and cook for another minute or two. Serve warm, drizzled with maple syrup and topped with nuts.

Free-Range Spring Apricot Chicken with Leeks

Fresh free-range chickens are abundant in spring and pairing them with leeks and plums creates a delicious complement.

SERVES 5 TO 7 | PREP TIME: 15 MINUTES | COOK TIME: 1 HOUR 30 MINUTES

- 1 (4 to 5 pounds) whole, organic, free-range chicken
- 2 tablespoons avocado oil, divided
- 1½ teaspoons sea salt, divided
- 2 cups thinly sliced leeks (white and light green part only)
- 1 tablespoon chopped fresh chives
- ¼ teaspoon ground pepper
- 3 apricots, pitted and halved
- ⅓ cup vegetable or chicken broth
- ¼ cup pine nuts (optional)

Preheat the oven to 375°F.

Pat the chicken very dry and place in a 9 × 13–inch baking dish. Rub with 1 tablespoon avocado oil and season with 1 teaspoon sea salt.

In a large bowl, combine the remaining 1 tablespoon oil, leeks, chives, pepper, and the remaining salt. Spread the leek mixture around the chicken in the baking dish. Add the apricots and broth. Roast for about 1 hour 20 minutes to 1 hour 30 minutes or until the chicken juices run clear and the temperature on a meat thermometer registers 165°F.

Remove from the oven and allow the chicken to rest for 20 to 25 minutes. Slice and serve topped with pine nuts if desired.

Chicken with Watercress Wraps

Turn your baked chicken into a chicken salad packed full of spring flavors. This recipe marries fresh herbs with seasonal greens and nuts, all wrapped up in tender collard greens. Ripe with flavor and nutrients!

SERVES 2 TO 3 | PREP TIME: 15 MINUTES | COOK TIME: 15 MINUTES

- 4 to 6 large collard greens, stemmed
- 2 tablespoons extra-virgin olive oil
- 1 tablespoon fresh lemon juice
- ¼ cup chopped fresh parsley
- 2 tablespoons chopped fresh mint
- 1 tablespoon chopped chives
- ½ teaspoon sea salt
- 1 pound cooked chicken breast, shredded (about 4 cups)
- 2 tablespoons chopped walnuts
- ¼ cup chopped green onions
- ½ cup watercress or microgreens

Bring a large pot of water to a simmer. Prepare an ice bath next to the stove. Once simmering, cook the collard greens leaves until they're bright green and softened, 10 to 15 seconds. Then immediately place them into the ice water to stop the cooking. Repeat with all of the leaves. Remove the leaves from the ice water, pat them dry, and set aside.

In a small bowl whisk together the olive oil, lemon juice, parsley, mint, chives, and salt. Set aside.

Combine the chicken, walnuts, green onions, and watercress in a large bowl. Drizzle around the olive oil mixture and toss to evenly coat.

Divide the chicken mixture among the collard greens leaves, placing it in the center of the leaf. Fold the short sides inward, then fold the bottom edge of the leaf over the top. Roll the wrap away from you like a jelly roll to seal. Repeat with the remaining wraps.

Creamy Artichoke Soup

Artichokes are rich in fiber and micronutrients like folate and vitamins A, C, and K. This creamy, delicious soup is gluten- and dairy-free and is packed full of antioxidants for glowing skin. Enjoy it warm in early spring and chilled in late spring.

SERVES 2 | PREP TIME: 10 MINUTES | COOK TIME: 25 MINUTES

- 1 tablespoon avocado oil
- 1 cup diced yellow onion
- 2 garlic cloves, minced
- 1 cup cauliflower florets
- 2 teaspoons fresh thyme leaves
- 2 cups organic free-range chicken broth or vegetable broth
- 1 (14-ounce) can artichokes in water, drained and rinsed
- 1 cup unsweetened plain almond milk
- ½ teaspoon sea salt
- 1 cup fresh organic spinach
- ⅓ cup chopped scallions
- Freshly ground pepper to taste

In a large saucepan, heat the avocado oil over medium heat. Sauté the onions and garlic until the onions are translucent, about 3 minutes.

Add the cauliflower and thyme, and sauté for another minute. Add the broth, artichokes, almond milk, and salt, and bring just to a boil. Reduce the heat to medium and simmer uncovered until the cauliflower is tender. Turn off the heat and stir in the spinach, allowing it to wilt.

Pour the soup into the carafe of a blender or food processor and purée on high speed until smooth and creamy. Divide into bowls and top with scallions and pepper to taste. Serve warm or cold.

Macadamia Nut Custard

This thick and creamy custard is the ultimate treat for spring when eggs are the freshest. The maple syrup adds mild sweetness, and the nuts on top add extra nutrients and flavor.

SERVES 3 TO 4 | PREP TIME: 10 MINUTES, PLUS 2 HOURS FOR CHILLING | COOK TIME: 10 MINUTES

- 5 large egg yolks
- ⅓ cup maple syrup
- 2 tablespoons tapioca flour
- 1 can full-fat coconut milk, well-shaken
- ½ teaspoon pure vanilla extract
- ¼ cup chopped raw macadamia nuts

In a medium-size bowl, whisk together the egg yolks, maple syrup, and tapioca flour, and set aside.

Heat the coconut milk in a medium-size saucepan over medium-low heat, stirring the milk occasionally with a wooden spoon until it starts to steam but not boil.

Remove the milk from the heat, and while whisking, gradually and slowly pour the milk into the egg mixture. Do not stop whisking as you add the coconut milk. Place the combined mixture back into the saucepan.

Heat the mixture over medium heat, whisking constantly until it starts to thicken like pudding and bubble, 2 to 3 minutes. Remove from the heat and whisk in the vanilla extract.

If there are any clumps, pour the custard through a strainer. Cover the custard and cool to room temperature and then refrigerate for at least 2 hours before serving. Serve cold topped with the chopped macadamia nuts.

Egg Dip with Veggies

Delicious and creamy with great flavor from the Dijon, vinegar, and chives, this B vitamin–rich dip pairs perfectly with fresh spring veggies like snap peas and radishes.

SERVES 3 TO 4 | PREP TIME: 10 MINUTES

- 6 hard-boiled eggs
- ¼ cup avocado mayonnaise
- 1 tablespoon Dijon mustard
- ½ tablespoon apple cider vinegar

– Sea salt and freshly ground black pepper pepper to taste

– 2 teaspoons chopped chives

– Radishes for dipping

– Snow or snap peas for dipping

Peel the shells from the boiled eggs and separate the egg whites from the yolks. Place the egg yolks in the bowl of a food processor fitted with the blade attachment. Chop the egg whites and place them in a medium bowl.

In the food processor, add the mayonnaise, mustard, and vinegar, and blend until smooth. Transfer the egg yolk mixture to the bowl with the whites. Season with salt, pepper, and chives, and stir to combine. Serve with radishes and snow peas.

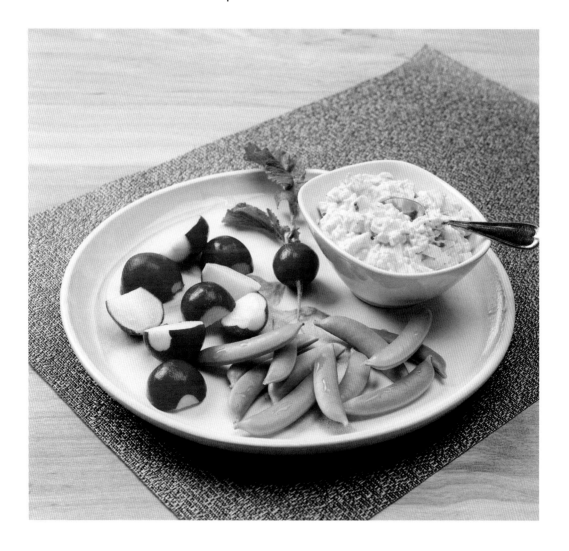

Strawberry Rhubarb Crisp

Tart and sweet is a sublime combination that you'll find in this tasty dessert. Topped with nuts instead of grains, and filled with fruit and maple syrup instead of sugar, you'll find this dessert easy on the belly and blood sugar.

SERVES 4 TO 6 | PREP TIME: 15 MINUTES | COOK TIME: 45 MINUTES

TOPPING:
– ¼ cup melted organic virgin coconut oil, plus extra for greasing the baking dish
– ½ cup almond flour
– ¼ cup chopped raw walnuts
– ¼ cup chopped raw macadamia nuts
– ¼ cup chopped raw cashews
– 1 tablespoon maple syrup
– Pinch sea salt

FILLING:
– 2 cups cut (¾-inch pieces) rhubarb
– 2 cups stemmed and cut (¾-inch pieces) strawberries
– ¼ cup maple syrup
– ½ teaspoon almond extract
– ½ teaspoon vanilla extract
– Pinch of sea salt

Preheat the oven to 350°F. Grease an 8 × 8–inch baking dish with coconut oil.

FOR THE TOPPING:
Combine the flour, walnuts, macadamia nuts, cashews, maple syrup, and salt, and mix until a crumbly texture forms. Set aside.

FOR THE FILLING:
In a separate large bowl, mix together the rhubarb, strawberries, maple syrup, almond extract, vanilla extract, and salt, and place the mixture into the baking dish. Evenly sprinkle the topping over the fruit mixture.

Bake for 40 to 45 minutes until the fruit is bubbly. Let cool for at least 15 minutes before serving.

Cherry Chocolate Mousse

Cherry and chocolate make an idyllic couple, and this dessert is no exception. Enjoy the sweetness while knowing you're nourishing your body with a healthy dose of antioxidants from the cherries and chocolate.

SERVES 2 TO 3 | PREP TIME: 15 MINUTES, PLUS CHILLING OVERNIGHT

- 1 (13.5-ounce) can full-fat coconut milk
- ⅛ cup unsweetened cocoa powder
- 1½ teaspoons monk fruit
- ½ teaspoon pure vanilla extract
- Pinch of sea salt
- ½ cup chopped fresh pitted cherries or thawed, drained, and chopped frozen dark, sweet cherries

Chill the can of coconut milk overnight in the refrigerator. About one hour before making, chill a metal bowl in the refrigerator as well.

Open the can of coconut milk and scoop out the solid portion at the top into the chilled bowl and discard the remaining liquid portion of the coconut milk.

Using an electric mixer, beat the coconut milk on high until whipped similar to cream, 5 to 8 minutes. Add the cocoa powder, monk fruit, vanilla, and salt, and whip again to combine.

Add the cherries and gently fold them into the mixture using a rubber spatula, and blend until incorporated. Serve immediately or freeze and serve cold.

Spring Onion Hummus with Nut Crackers

Dip into this creamy spring dip and discover the fresh flavors of garlic, onion, and cumin. Pair with Nut Crackers for the perfect duo.

2 CUPS | PREP TIME: 10 MINUTES

- 1 (15-ounce) can garbanzo beans, drained and rinsed, or 1½ cups cooked garbanzo beans
- 2 tablespoons extra-virgin olive oil
- ¼ cup well-stirred tahini
- 1 lemon, juiced
- ¼ cup spring onions or scallions
- 1 green garlic stalk
- ½ teaspoon ground cumin
- ½ teaspoon sea salt
- 5 tablespoons to ½ cup hot water

In a food processor fitted with the blade attachment, combine the garbanzo beans, olive oil, tahini, lemon juice, spring onions, green garlic, cumin, and salt. Pulse until a smooth consistency forms. Start with less water and continue adding water as necessary until a very smooth texture forms. Move to an airtight container and refrigerate until ready to use. Serve with Nut Crackers (see recipe on page 188). Store the dip in an airtight container in the refrigerator for up to three days.

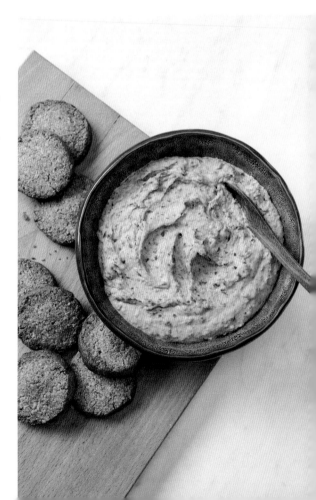

SUMMER RECIPES

Peach Coconut Mint Smoothie

Summer is flourishing and full of flavor, which you'll find in this fresh and delicious peach and coconut smoothie with mint. The fiber and antioxidants help harmonize your blood sugar and hormones for a fabulous start to your day!

SERVES 1 | PREP TIME: 5 MINUTES

- 1 cup unsweetened coconut milk
- ½ cup fresh peaches, pitted and chopped, or frozen peaches
- ½ cup ice (skip if using frozen peaches)
- ⅓ cup fresh or dried unsweetened flaked coconut
- ½ cup summer greens
- 7 mint leaves
- 1 tablespoon crushed raw macadamia nuts
- 1 dash stevia powder (optional)

In a blender, combine the coconut milk, peaches, ice (if using), flaked coconut, greens, mint, macadamia nuts, and stevia, and blend until smooth. Pour the mixture into a tall glass and enjoy cold.

Berry Bliss Smoothie Bowl

Summer is the season of berries, and pairing them with avocado and coconut milk balances the carbs for the ideal breakfast smoothie bowl.

SERVES 1 | PREP TIME: 5 MINUTES

- ½ cup unsweetened full-fat coconut milk
- ½ cup fresh berries
- ¼ cup ice
- ½ cup summer greens
- ½ ripe avocado, peeled and pitted
- 5 to 6 basil leaves
- 1 dash stevia powder (optional)
- 1 tablespoon coconut flakes, toasted for garnish
- ¼ cup fresh berries, for garnish

Combine the coconut milk, fresh berries, ice, summer greens, avocado, basil, and stevia if desired in the carafe of a high-speed blender. Blend until smooth, stirring periodically (the mixture will be very thick). Cover and chill if desired. Pour into a bowl and top with the coconut flakes and berries.

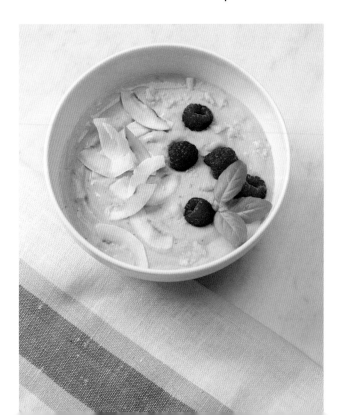

Green Goddess Smoothie

Nourish your inner goddess with this very veggie and berry smoothie.

SERVES 1 | PREP TIME: 5 MINUTES

- ½ cup chilled chamomile tea
- ¼ cup fresh or frozen berries
- ¼ cup chopped and unpeeled cucumber
- ¼ cup ice (skip if using frozen berries)
- ½ tablespoon spirulina or chlorella powder
- ½ cup summer greens
- ¼ avocado, pitted and peeled
- 1 dash stevia powder (optional)

In a blender, combine the tea, berries, cucumber, ice (if using), spirulina, greens, avocado, and stevia if desired, and blend until smooth. Pour into a glass and enjoy. Chill before drinking if desired.

Golden Mango Smoothie

Create a summer escape with the tropical flavors of mango, coconut, and turmeric. Add in maca for an extra energy boost.

SERVES 1 | PREP TIME: 5 MINUTES

- 1 cup organic unsweetened coconut milk
- ⅓ cup unsweetened organic coconut flakes
- ⅓ cup peeled and pitted fresh mango or frozen mango chunks
- ½ teaspoon ground turmeric
- ¼ cup ice cubes made from filtered water
- 1 dash stevia powder (optional)
- ½ teaspoon dried maca (optional)

In a blender, combine the coconut milk, coconut flakes, mango, turmeric, ice, and stevia and maca if desired, and blend until smooth. Pour into a tall glass and enjoy cold.

Wild Alaskan Salmon with Pesto Green Beans

Wild Alaskan salmon is easier to find fresh in summer so enjoy it with your favorite produce such as the green beans in this recipe. We boost the flavor and nutritional content with fresh herb pesto.

SERVES 4 | PREP TIME: 15 MINUTES | COOK TIME: 20 MINUTES

SALMON AND GREEN BEANS:
- 1 pound wild Alaskan salmon fillets
- 1 tablespoon avocado oil
- 1 tablespoon lemon juice
- ¼ teaspoon sea salt
- Freshly ground black pepper
- 1 pound green beans, ends trimmed

BASIL PESTO:
- ½ cup pine nuts
- 2 cups fresh basil, packed
- 3 garlic cloves
- ½ teaspoon sea salt
- ½ lemon, juiced
- ½ cup extra-virgin olive oil

FOR THE SALMON AND GREEN BEANS:

Preheat the oven to 400°F. Line a baking sheet with parchment paper.

Rub the salmon with avocado oil and season to taste with lemon juice, salt, and pepper. Place in a baking dish, and bake for 15 to 18 minutes or until firm, opaque, and cooked through.

Bring an inch of water to a boil in a large pot fitted with a steamer basket. Add the green beans, cover, and steam for 5 to 7 minutes (until tender/crisp). Move to a medium bowl and set aside.

FOR THE PESTO:

Add the pine nuts, basil, garlic, salt, and lemon juice to the bowl of a food processor. Pulse until finely chopped. While the machine is running, slowly drizzle in the olive oil and pulse until smooth and combined.

Pour half of the pesto over the green beans, and toss until evenly coated. Serve the salmon with the green beans and extra pesto on the side.

Watermelon Salad with Mint and Goat Feta

What fruit screams summer more than watermelon? Enjoy fresh summer flavors of feta, watermelon, and mint for a sweet-and-salty combination packed with lycopene, vitamin C, and vitamin A. Goat feta is easier to find fresh and is generally more flavorful in summer, so it's an excellent addition, but if you're dairy intolerant, you can skip it.

SERVES 4 | PREP TIME: 15 MINUTES

- 5 cups 1-inch cubed seedless watermelon, chilled
- 1 cup diced English cucumber
- ¼ cup minced fresh mint leaves
- 2 tablespoons extra-virgin olive oil
- 2 tablespoons minced shallots
- Pinch sea salt (or more to taste)
- 2 cups arugula
- 2 ounces goat feta, crumbled
- ½ cup macadamia nuts, chopped (optional)

In a large bowl, combine the watermelon, cucumber, mint, olive oil, shallots, and salt. Add the arugula, feta, and macadamia nuts if desired, and gently toss to combine. Serve chilled.

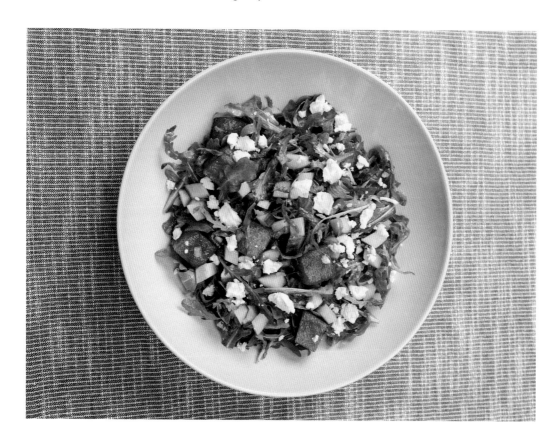

Summer Greens Salad with Black-Eyed Peas

Relish the sun-loving greens paired with sweet summer tomatoes and topped with fiber-and-protein-rich black-eyed peas for a southern twist to this seasonal salad.

SERVES 3 TO 4 | PREP TIME: 15 MINUTES

- 1 (15-ounce) can black-eyed peas, drained and rinsed
- ¾ cup ripe tomato, diced
- 1 shallot, minced
- 2 tablespoons chopped fresh cilantro
- 2 tablespoons chopped fresh basil
- 1 tablespoon apple cider vinegar
- 1 teaspoon Dijon mustard
- 3 tablespoons extra-virgin olive oil
- Sea salt to taste
- Freshly ground pepper to taste
- 6 cups summer greens

In a large bowl, combine the black-eyed peas with the tomato, shallot, cilantro, basil, vinegar, mustard, oil, salt, and pepper, and gently toss to combine.

Divide the greens among four plates and top with the black-eyed pea salad.

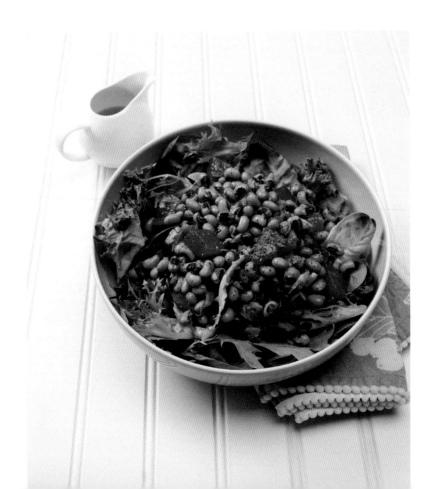

Lamb Chops with Mint Chutney

Lamb is generally easier to find fresh and known for its best flavors in summer, so it's the ideal time to put it on the grill or in a cast-iron skillet. Coupled with mint, it's the perfect summer flavorful dish with a boost in zinc, vitamin B$_{12}$, iron, and protein.

SERVES 4 TO 5 | PREP TIME: 10 MINUTES, PLUS 30 MINUTES TO 4 HOURS FOR MARINATING | COOK TIME: 15 MINUTES

LAMB CHOPS:

- 2 green garlic stalks, trimmed and minced
- 2 teaspoons sea salt
- ¼ teaspoon freshly ground black pepper
- 3 tablespoons avocado oil, divided
- 8 (4-ounce) lamb chops

MINT CHUTNEY:

- ½ cup fresh mint leaves
- 1 cup parsley, leaves and stems
- 1 green garlic stalk, trimmed and minced, or 2 regular garlic cloves, minced
- ½ teaspoon sea salt
- Freshly ground black pepper to taste
- 2 teaspoons apple cider vinegar
- ¼ cup extra-virgin olive oil

FOR THE LAMB CHOPS:

In a small bowl, combine the green garlic, salt, pepper, and 1 tablespoon of the oil.

Coat the chops with the marinade and allow to marinate for 30 minutes at room temperature or covered in the fridge for up to 4 hours.

FOR THE CHUTNEY:

Place the mint, parsley, and garlic in the bowl of a food processor fitted with the blade attachment. Add the salt, pepper, vinegar, and olive oil, and pulse all of the ingredients until they make a sauce.

Heat a large heavy-bottomed skillet or cast-iron skillet over medium heat and add 1 tablespoon of oil to coat the pan. Add the lamb chops in a single layer. Cook until browned, about 3 to 4 minutes, on each side (for medium-rare to medium chops).

Serve the lamb warm topped with the mint chutney.

Macadamia-Crusted Trout with Pineapple Chutney

Fresh-caught trout is easier to find in summer, and this macadamia nut–crusted recipe is topped with a delicious pineapple chutney full of bromelain and flavor!

SERVES 4 | PREP TIME: 15 MINUTES | COOK TIME: 15 MINUTES

PINEAPPLE CHUTNEY:
- ½ cup fresh pineapple chunks
- ¼ cup roughly chopped English cucumber
- 2 tablespoons roughly chopped shallots
- 2 tablespoons fresh cilantro
- ½ teaspoon extra-virgin olive oil

MACADAMIA-CRUSTED TROUT:
- ½ cup finely chopped dry roasted macadamia nuts
- ½ cup almond flour
- ½ cup flaked or shredded unsweetened coconut
- 1 tablespoon chopped fresh cilantro
- 1 tablespoon chopped fresh parsley
- ½ teaspoon sea salt, plus more to taste
- Freshly ground black pepper to taste
- 2 large egg whites or 1 tablespoon agar plus 2 tablespoons water or ½ teaspoon xanthan gum plus ½ teaspoon water
- 4 (2 pounds) trout fillets, skin removed
- 2 tablespoons avocado oil, plus more as needed

FOR THE CHUTNEY:
In a food processor, add the pineapple, cucumber, shallots, cilantro, and olive oil, and pulse until finely chopped. Chill or serve at room temperature.

FOR THE TROUT:
Combine the macadamia nuts, almond flour, coconut, cilantro, parsley, salt, and pepper in a shallow dish. In another dish, lightly whisk the egg whites until frothy.

Pat the fish dry and dip them into the egg whites and then coat the fish with the nut mixture.

Heat the avocado oil in a large skillet over medium-high heat and add half the fish fillets in a single layer. Cook until golden and the fish is opaque and flaky, about 2 to 3 minutes per side. Repeat with the remaining fish fillets. Top with the pineapple chutney and serve.

Summer Gazpacho

As my grandmother used to say, "it's not summer until you've had a fresh bowl of gazpacho." This fresh and herb-enhanced gazpacho is packed with antioxidants like lycopene. I can see grandmother smiling!

SERVES 2 TO 4 | PREP TIME: 10 MINUTES, PLUS CHILLING TIME

- 6 ripe tomatoes, halved and cored
- 2 small cucumbers, peeled, seeded, and chopped
- ½ yellow or red onion, chopped
- 2 tablespoons fresh parsley leaves
- 2 tablespoons chopped fresh chives, plus additional for garnish
- 2 cloves garlic, minced
- ½ large shallot, chopped
- 2 tablespoons apple cider vinegar
- ¼ cup extra-virgin olive oil
- 1 teaspoon sea salt
- ½ teaspoon freshly ground pepper
- ½ avocado, pitted and peeled, plus more diced for garnish

Place the tomatoes, cucumbers, onion, parsley, chives, garlic, shallot, vinegar, oil, salt, pepper, and avocado in the bowl of a food processor fitted with the blade attachment and purée for 1 minute or until the soup reaches the desired consistency. Refrigerate in a glass container with a lid for 3 hours or until chilled. Serve chilled topped with diced avocado and minced chives.

Cucumber Salad

Cucumbers are both hydrating and refreshing, making them the perfect summer veggie. Mixed with radishes, fresh mint, and parsley, this is a cooling dish for hot summer days.

SERVES 2 | PREP TIME: 15 MINUTES

- 2 cups cubed organic English cucumber
- 1 cup thinly sliced radishes
- ¼ cup chopped parsley
- 3 tablespoons chopped mint
- 3 green garlic stalks or scallions, minced
- 2 tablespoons apple cider vinegar
- 2 tablespoons extra-virgin olive oil
- ¼ teaspoon sea salt
- 4 cups summer greens, such as arugula

In a large bowl, combine the cucumber, radishes, parsley, mint, garlic, vinegar, oil, salt, and greens, and toss gently to combine. Serve chilled or at room temperature.

Tomato and Peach Summer Salad

Although it may seem like an unlikely combination, tomatoes and peaches are divine together, especially when topped with fresh corn and a seasonal herbal dressing. Antioxidants and flavors are copious in this salad.

SERVES 3 TO 4 | PREP TIME: 15 MINUTES

- 2 tablespoons extra-virgin olive oil
- 1 tablespoon apple cider vinegar
- ½ tablespoon Dijon mustard
- ½ shallot, minced
- 2 tablespoons fresh mint leaves
- ¼ cup fresh parsley leaves
- Sea salt to taste
- Freshly ground black pepper to taste
- ¾ cup fresh corn kernels, cut from the cob
- 2 medium ripe tomatoes, cut into wedges
- 2 medium peaches, pitted and cut into wedges
- 4 radishes, thinly sliced
- 1 cup purslane, chopped (use arugula or spinach if purslane is not available)
- 4 ounces goat feta, crumbled

In a large bowl, whisk together the olive oil, vinegar, mustard, shallot, mint, parsley, salt, and pepper. Add the corn, tomatoes, peaches, radishes, and purslane and toss to coat. Season to taste with salt and pepper and top with goat feta.

Summer Squash Tacos

These tacos have no meat, but they're so filling and full of flavor that you won't miss it. Enjoy the summer squash and avocado sauce with collard greens or corn tortillas. You can make your own or try to find a fresh source at a local market.

SERVES 3 TO 4 | PREP TIME: 20 MINUTES | COOK TIME: 15 MINUTES

AVOCADO SAUCE:
- ⅓ cup cilantro
- 2 ripe avocados, pitted, sliced into chunks, and skin removed
- 1 clove garlic
- 1 tablespoon apple cider vinegar
- 1 tablespoon extra-virgin olive oil
- 1 tablespoon water
- Sea salt and black pepper to taste
- 1 cup chopped ripe tomato

SQUASH FILLING:
- 2 tablespoons extra-virgin olive oil
- ½ shallot, chopped

- 2 (8 ounces) medium summer squashes (zucchini and yellow squash), chopped
- ½ teaspoon chili powder (optional)
- ¼ teaspoon ground cumin
- 1 ear of corn, husked and kernels sliced off the cob
- 1 cup sliced cherry tomatoes
- ½ teaspoon sea salt
- Freshly ground black pepper to taste
- 1 15-ounce can black-eyed peas
- 6 small non-GMO organic corn tortillas
- ½ cup thinly sliced radishes

FOR THE AVOCADO SAUCE:

In the bowl of a food processor fitted with the blade attachment, blend the cilantro, avocado, garlic, and vinegar. Add the olive oil and water, season with salt and pepper, and pulse again until very smooth. Use a spatula to transfer to a small bowl and stir in the tomato. Set aside.

FOR THE SQUASH FILLING:

Heat the oil in a large skillet over medium heat. Add the shallot and cook for 2 minutes until translucent. Then add the squash, chili powder, cumin, corn, tomatoes, salt, and black pepper. Cook for 5 minutes, stirring occasionally, or until the squash is crisp-tender.

Reduce to low heat and stir in the black-eyed peas. Cook until just heated through, about 3 minutes. Remove from the heat.

Over medium heat in a small skillet, heat each tortilla on each side for about 5 to 10 seconds or until warmed.

Place the squash filling in the middle of each tortilla, and top with avocado sauce and sliced radishes.

Ratatouille

Everything you need to make this classic dish is abundant in summer. If you have a garden, you may be wondering what to make with all the extra squash and zucchini, and here's your answer! Take your time and let this cook and soak in the flavors, and enjoy!

SERVES 3 TO 4 | PREP TIME: 15 MINUTES | COOK TIME: 1 HOUR 45 MINUTES

- 2 (1 pound) medium eggplants
- 2 (8 ounces) yellow squashes
- 2 (8 ounces) zucchinis
- 2 tablespoons avocado oil
- Sea salt to taste
- Freshly ground black pepper to taste
- 2 large ripe tomatoes
- ½ cup vegetable broth
- ¼ cup chopped fresh basil
- 2 tablespoons chopped fresh parsley
- Olive oil for drizzle finish

Preheat the oven to 350°F. Line two baking sheets with parchment paper.

Slice the eggplants, squashes, and zucchinis into ¼-inch-thick rounds. Place them on the prepared baking sheets and drizzle with avocado oil. Season with salt and pepper to taste and toss to evenly coat. Roast for 40 to 45 minutes until softened, flipping halfway through.

Meanwhile, bring a large pot of water to boil for the tomatoes. Score an X on the bottom of the tomatoes using a paring knife. Place them in the boiling water to blanch, about 10 to 20 seconds, then remove and place them in cold water. Remove the skin and seeds and discard. Roughly chop the tomatoes.

Add the prepared veggies to a large pot with vegetable broth. Allow to simmer over medium-low heat for 20 to 30 minutes until the vegetables are broken down and very tender. Stir in the basil and parsley and season again with salt and pepper to taste. Serve warm with additional herbs and a drizzle of oil.

SNACKS AND DESSERTS

Coconut Ice Cream

Most of us grew up believing it's just not summer without ice cream. I used to have to pass on ice cream because I couldn't tolerate the dairy, but then I discovered my own recipe using coconut milk. It's so simple, delicious, sweet, and creamy. Now we all get to enjoy it.

SERVES 3 TO 4 | PREP TIME: 5 MINUTES, PLUS 12 HOURS FOR FREEZING

– 1 can full-fat coconut milk

– ½ cup honey

– Pinch of sea salt

– 1 teaspoon pure vanilla extract

In a bowl, whisk together the coconut milk, honey, salt, and vanilla until smooth and well combined. Portion into ice cube trays and freeze until softly frozen, about 8 hours. Once softly frozen, blend in a high-powered blender. Place into a 9 × 5–inch loaf pan and allow to freeze again for at least 4 hours. Serve.

Creamy Chocolate Mousse Parfait

This creamy dessert has a surprising ingredient—avocados! Don't let that deter you because it creates a creamy texture that will thrill your taste buds, and your body will love the extra antioxidants and monounsaturated fats to support your hormonal harmony.

SERVES 3 TO 4 | PREP TIME: 5 MINUTES

- 2 ripe avocados, pitted and peeled
- ¼ cup unsweetened pure cocoa powder
- ¼ cup honey
- ½ cup full-fat coconut milk, well-shaken
- 2 teaspoons pure vanilla extract
- Pinch sea salt
- ½ cup berries (or other summer fruit)
- ¼ cup raw macadamia nuts
- ¼ cup shredded unsweetened coconut

In a food processor, blend the avocados until smooth and then add the cocoa powder, honey, coconut milk, vanilla, and salt. Blend until smooth.

Move to an airtight container and refrigerate for 30 minutes to 1 hour.

Create parfaits by alternately layering the chocolate mousse, berries, nuts, and coconut. Serve immediately.

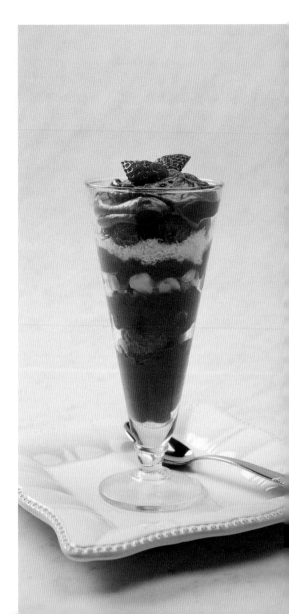

Summer Berry Crisp

I have many fond memories picking wild berries in the summers and turning them into homemade berry crisp. With this recipe, we're swapping out the sugar, butter, and wheat flour for a healthier version that is just as tasty!

SERVES 6 | PREP TIME: 10 MINUTES | COOK TIME: 45 MINUTES

TOPPING:

- 2 tablespoons melted organic virgin coconut oil, plus extra for greasing
- ½ cup almond flour
- ½ cup unsweetened coconut flakes
- ½ cup chopped raw macadamia nuts
- 3 tablespoon raw honey
- Pinch of sea salt

FILLING:

- 4 cups fresh berries
- 1 teaspoon vanilla extract
- Dash of stevia (optional)

Preheat the oven to 350°F. Grease an 8 × 8–inch baking dish with coconut oil.

FOR THE TOPPING:

In a medium bowl, stir together the oil, flour, coconut flakes, macadamia nuts, honey, and salt until crumbly. Set aside.

FOR THE FILLING:

In a large bowl, mix the berries, vanilla, and stevia if desired together, and pour into the baking dish. Sprinkle the topping evenly over the berry mixture.

Bake for 40 to 45 minutes until the fruit is bubbly and the topping is golden brown. Allow to cool for 15 minutes and serve warm topped with Coconut Ice Cream (see recipe).

Roasted Tomatillo Salsa

Enjoy a fresh salsa full of flavor, lycopene, and vitamin C to nourish your skin from within. Serve with tacos or make your own non-GMO corn or cassava chips.

SERVES 4 TO 6 | **PREP TIME: 10 MINUTES** | **COOK TIME: 20 MINUTES**

- 2 ripe tomatoes, halved
- 5 tomatillos, husked and halved
- ½ shallot, roughly chopped
- ⅓ small red onion, roughly chopped
- ½ cup chopped cilantro
- 1 teaspoon apple cider vinegar or lime juice
- Sea salt and freshly ground black pepper to taste

Preheat the oven to 400°F. Line a baking sheet with parchment paper.

Place the tomatoes and tomatillos cut-side down onto the baking sheet. Roast for 20 minutes until very tender.

Place the tomatoes and tomatillos into the bowl of a food processor fitted with the blade attachment. Add the shallot, onion, cilantro, and vinegar, and blend until smooth. Season with salt and pepper to taste. Serve with organic corn chips or over greens with black-eyed peas.

Melon with Coconut Sauce

So fresh and tropical tasting, this recipe can be enjoyed as a breakfast, snack, or dessert.

SERVES 4 | **PREP TIME: 15 MINUTES, PLUS 30 MINUTES FOR CHILLING**
COOK TIME: 5 MINUTES

- 1 cup full-fat coconut milk, well-shaken
- 1 teaspoon raw honey
- 1 teaspoon tapioca flour
- 1 teaspoon vanilla extract
- 5 to 6 cups melon balls or diced melon (watermelon, honeydew, or cantaloupe)
- ½ cup shredded sweetened coconut
- ¼ cup chopped fresh mint

In a small saucepan, combine the coconut milk, honey, and flour. Simmer over medium heat whisking constantly until slightly thickened, about 5 minutes. Remove from the heat, stir in the vanilla extract, and chill in the refrigerator for 30 minutes.

Divide and place the melon balls into four dishes, then drizzle with coconut mixture. Sprinkle with the shredded coconut and garnish with the mint.

DIY SKINCARE RECIPES

The DIY skincare recipes in this chapter are designed to provide natural at-home solutions for your skin during the seven-day reset for each season. For long-term daily skincare, I suggest using a high-quality natural skincare line such as The Spa Dr.'s Daily Essentials.

DIY SKINCARE TIPS

- Use these recipes when they're fresh. Since they do not contain preservatives, they will not last more than a few days, even when refrigerated.
- Some ingredients can grow bacteria and mold quickly, while other natural ingredients have antioxidant and antimicrobial properties that help keep the formula fresh.
- Even though they're all-natural ingredients, it is possible for some people to have allergic reactions and skin irritation. It's best to do a skin patch test before using products. To do this, apply on the inside of your wrist, and, for the next few hours, watch for any redness, swelling, or irritation. If you have a reaction, avoid the product.
- If you're aware of an allergy to any of the ingredients when you eat them, do not put them on your face.
- Store these DIY recipes in a jar or tightly sealed glass container in the refrigerator to preserve freshness.
- Avoid over exfoliation—recipes for the face should feel smooth, not rough.

FALL DIY

Chia, Honey, and Green Tea Face Wash

Step into fall with a clean slate using this antioxidant-packed DIY face wash. Green tea is rich in antioxidants that help soothe, protect, and brighten the skin. When mixed with liquid, chia seeds turn into a gel, giving the recipes texture and thickness. Honey contains enzymes to help cleanse and gently exfoliate.

MAKES ABOUT 4 APPLICATIONS

– 1 tablespoon chia seeds

– ¼ cup distilled water

– 2 teaspoons brewed and chilled jasmine green tea

– 1½ tablespoons organic raw honey

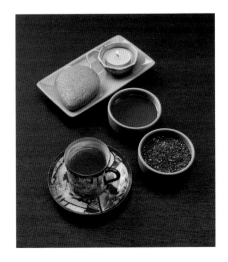

In a small bowl, soak the chia seeds in distilled water for 10 minutes. Meanwhile, brew green tea by adding 1 tea bag to 8 ounces of hot water and letting it steep for 3 minutes. Add the warm tea and honey to the soaked chia seeds. Usually, the chia seeds will have soaked up all the water, but if not, any remaining water from soaking can be strained off. Allow to cool to room temperature before applying to your face.

Apply about 1 tablespoon of mixture to your face in circular motions and rinse with cool water. Store the unused portion in a closed container in the refrigerator. Use within three days.

Herbal Face Steam

Create an herbal infusion with dried sunflower petals and chamomile flowers to hydrate and nourish your skin. While this is a practice to enjoy all year, this blend uses fall herbs to help soothe skin during cooler days.

MAKES 1 APPLICATION

– ⅓ cup dried sunflower petals

– ⅓ cup dried calendula blossoms

– 2 cups filtered water for steeping, plus extra for steam

– 4 to 5 drops lavender essential oil

Add the dried sunflower and calendula to a large French press or teapot. Boil the water and pour it over the flowers and steep for about 10 minutes.

Fill a large pot halfway with very hot water. Press or strain the flowers, then add the infusion to the hot water. Add the lavender oil.

Pull up a chair that will allow you to hang your head over the pot, about 6 to 8 inches from the water. Drape a large bath towel over your head and shoulders to create a tent over the pot, and steam your face and neck for 3 to 5 minutes. Add hot water as needed to produce more steam. After steaming, wash with a DIY cleanser (such as the Chia, Honey, and Green Tea Face Wash) and pat dry with a clean, soft towel. Discard the water and herbs after use.

Pumpkin Face Mask

Pumpkin contains enzymes that naturally brighten and exfoliate. Oats are soothing and calming, and honey is a natural humectant. This powerhouse list of fall ingredients provides the nourishment your skin needs for cooler, drier days ahead.

MAKES ABOUT 3 TO 4 APPLICATIONS

- 2 tablespoons rolled oats
- 1 teaspoon raw honey
- 1 tablespoon cooked pumpkin (make your own or use canned)
- 1 teaspoon plain kefir or raw whole milk

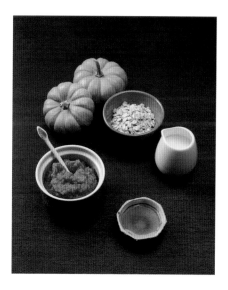

Soak the oats for 5 minutes, allowing the oats to gel a bit, which increases the soothing and humectant benefits. Place the oats, honey, pumpkin, and kefir in a food processor and blend until smooth.

Apply about 1 tablespoon of the mask to a clean, dry face. Leave on for 5 to 10 minutes, and then rinse off with warm water. Store in a closed container in the refrigerator, and use within 3 days.

WINTER DIY

Cleansing Body Oil

Hydrate dry winter skin while cleansing with this nourishing blend of plant-based oils. Sweet almond oil is high in essential fatty acids so it helps protect skin's barrier function, keeping it soft and moisturized. Castor oil is cleansing, avocado oil adds extra nourishment, and the fresh scent of oranges brightens your winter day.

MAKES 3 TO 5 APPLICATIONS

- 1 tablespoon sweet almond oil
- 1 tablespoon castor oil
- 3 tablespoons avocado oil
- 3 drops orange essential oil

In a jar, mix together the almond, castor, avocado, and orange oils.

When ready to use, apply 1 to 2 tablespoons to your entire body and then step into a warm shower. Enjoy your shower and use this oil as your cleanser instead of using a bar of soap or body wash, which have a high pH and strip the skin of natural oils. When you get out of the shower or bath, pat, don't rub, your skin dry so you don't remove all of those fabulous oils. Keep the jar closed and store in a cool, dry, dark place. Use within six months.

Winter Body Scrub

Scrub those winter blues away with an invigorating body scrub. Enjoy the hydration from the almond oil and natural exfoliation from the coffee and cane sugar. Allow the spearmint essential oil to lift your spirits as you exfoliate dry skin.

MAKES 2 TO 3 APPLICATIONS

- ½ cup jojoba or sweet almond oil
- 1 cup pure fine cane sugar
- ½ cup freshly used coffee grounds
- 5 to 10 drops spearmint essential oil (skip if you have sensitive skin)

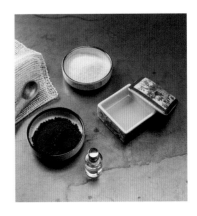

In a bowl, combine the jojoba, sugar, coffee grounds, and spearmint oil, then transfer to a wide-mouthed jar, and store in a cool place until ready to use.

In the shower, apply handfuls of the scrub to wet skin in circular motions, starting at the feet and working up. Spend extra time on rough spots such as knees, elbows, heels, and ankles.

This recipe is for use as a body scrub, not a facial scrub. Keep your application below the neck, and do not apply to any sensitive areas. Store unused portions in a closed container in the refrigerator. Use within three days.

Soothing Lip Balm

Prevent chapped lips and achieve seductively soft lips with this natural lip balm. Swap out the mineral oil and petroleum-based synthetic lip products this winter for this plant-based nourishing blend.

MAKES 4 TABLESPOONS

- 1 tablespoon cocoa butter
- 2 tablespoons shea butter
- 1 tablespoon coconut oil
- 7 to 14 drops vanilla or spearmint essential oil
- Lip balm tins or small jars

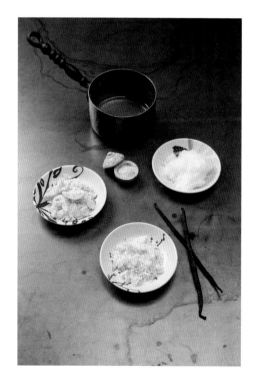

In a small pot over low-medium heat, melt the cocoa butter, shea butter, and coconut oil. Remove from the heat and quickly add the essential oil to make sure it is fully incorporated before the mixture hardens. Whisk together well. Once blended and still in liquid form, quickly pour it into tins or jars. Let cool in the refrigerator until it hardens.

During cool weather, the balm can be stored at room temperature. During warm weather, store in the refrigerator. Apply liberally as needed to lips. Keep the container closed, and store in a cool, dry, dark place. Use within six months.

SPRING DIY

Spring Face Oil

Spring into warmer months with naturally hydrated skin. Your face (and mind) will thank you for this nourishing blend. Use jojoba oil as a base since it's light and great for all skin types, including oily skin, and add one to four of the essential oils below.

MAKES 1 OUNCE

– 1 ounce jojoba oil

– Essential oil blend. Choose from any of the following:

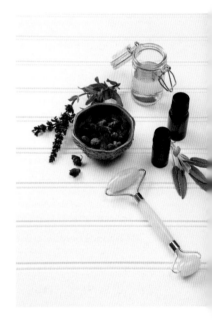

- Geranium
- Jasmine
- Lavender
- Bergamot
- Clary sage
- Rose
- May chang
- Ylang-ylang
- Neroli
- Rosewood

Place jojoba oil in an amber or cobalt blue glass bottle, either with a pump, dropper top, or orifice reducer. Select one to four of your favorite essential oils from the list above. Add 3 to 6 drops of the oil blend to the jojoba oil.

Apply a few drops to clean skin and gently massage into your face and neck. Avoid the eye area. Keep the container closed, and store in a cool, dry, dark place. Use within a year.

Face Refresher

After the winter months, our skin often feels dull, and this DIY face recipe is the perfect solution to revitalize tired dry skin. Egg whites* are known for their ability to tone skin, while green peas brighten and yogurt balances.

MAKES ABOUT 4 APPLICATIONS

– 1 egg white*

– 4 tablespoons cooked green peas

– 2 tablespoons unsweetened whole Greek yogurt

In a food processor, blend together the egg white, peas, and yogurt until smooth.

Apply about 1 tablespoon to a clean, dry face. Keep out of the eye area and away from the mouth. Leave on for 5 minutes and then rinse off with warm water. Discard unused portion and make fresh with each use.

---

*Always use caution with raw eggs since they can be contaminated with the harmful bacteria salmonella and cause food poisoning if ingested.

Strawberry and Apricot Face Mask

Infuse your skin with fresh spring produce full of nourishing antioxidants. Apricots and strawberries are in season, so enjoy their freshness along with hydrating jojoba oil and dandelion tea. Adding in bentonite clay helps purify skin and balance its natural oils.

MAKES 6 APPLICATIONS

- 4 strawberries
- 1 small apricot, halved and pitted
- ½ tablespoon jojoba oil
- 1½ teaspoons dandelion flower tea or other spring herb tea
- 2 teaspoons bentonite clay

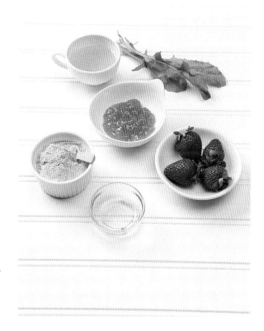

In a food processor, blend the strawberries, apricot, oil, and tea into a smooth pulp. Move the pulp to a small bowl and mix in the clay to form a thicker consistency.

Apply about 1 tablespoon of the mask to a clean, damp face. Let it sit for 10 to 15 minutes. Rinse gently with lukewarm water. Store unused portion in a closed container in the refrigerator. Use within three days.

SUMMER DIY

Cucumber Mint Face Mist

Revive skin and cool off from the summer heat with this refreshing face mist. Cucumber's soothing and hydrating properties along with the cleansing and toning benefits of mint make this the perfect summertime DIY recipe.

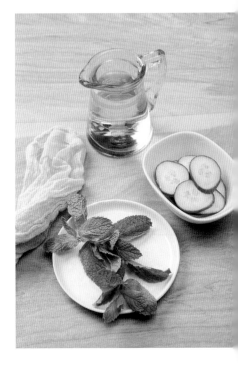

MAKES ENOUGH FOR A 4- TO 6-OUNCE SPRAY BOTTLE

- ½ cup distilled water
- 4 mint leaves
- ½ cucumber
- 1 cheese cloth
- 4 to 6 ounce spray bottle

In a food processor, blend the distilled water, mint, and cucumber, and then press the mixture through cheese cloth. Place the strained mixture in a spray bottle. Shake vigorously and spritz your face two to three times per use. Store unused portion in a closed container in the refrigerator. Use within three days.

Jojoba Oil and Yogurt Cleanser

Summer heat can trigger breakouts and clogged pores, which means it's time to focus on cleansing while balancing oils on your skin. This natural DIY cleanser is good for all skin types, including those with combination and oily skin.

MAKES ABOUT 6 APPLICATIONS (3 TABLESPOONS)

- 2 tablespoons avocado
- 2 teaspoons jojoba oil
- 2 tablespoons unsweetened organic Greek yogurt

In a food processor, blend together the avocado, oil, and yogurt.

Apply ½ tablespoon to your face, gently massage it for 1 to 2 minutes, and then rinse with warm water. Store unused portions in a closed container in the refrigerator. Use within three days.

Hydrating Watermelon Face Mask

The secret to glowing skin in summer is hydration and balance, which is precisely what you'll find with this DIY mask. Watermelon provides an excellent source of the antioxidant lycopene, and this juicy fruit is packed with hydration benefits. Bentonite helps relieve congested skin, and yogurt contains enzymes and active cultures that help quell inflammation and balance skin's pH for a healthy skin microbiome.

MAKES ENOUGH FOR 5 APPLICATIONS

- ¼ cup chopped watermelon
- 1 teaspoon organic honey
- 3 tablespoons plain unsweetened yogurt
- 1 tablespoon bentonite or French green clay

In a food processor, purée the watermelon, then add the honey and yogurt until fully blended. Transfer to a small bowl and mix in the clay to thicken the consistency.

Apply ½ tablespoon of the mixture evenly to clean, dry skin. Leave on your face for 10 to 15 minutes, then rinse with warm water. Store in a closed container in the refrigerator. Use within three days.

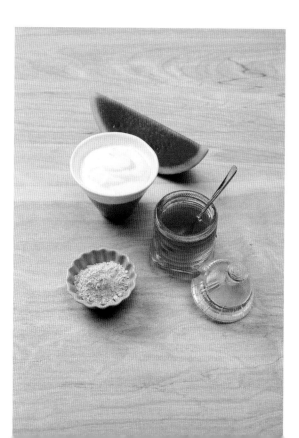

RESOURCES

In this section, I will include resources mentioned throughout the book to complement the 7-Day Natural Beauty Reset.

For an online quiz to help you customize the Natural Beauty Reset to meet your unique needs, visit www.TheSpaDr.com/Quiz.

For natural skincare options, visit www.TheSpaDr.com/skincare.

For supplement ideas and options, visit www.TheSpaDr.com/supplements.

For recommendations to complement and enhance the program, visit www.TheSpaDr.com/referrals.

For more on the link between skincare and hormones, visit www.TheSpaDr.com/hormones.

For more about the *Hormones, Health, and Harmony* docuseries, visit www.TheWomansDr.com/docuseries.

For more seasonal food recommendations, go to the Seasonal Food Guide at www.seasonalfoodguide.org.[178] Visit your local farmers market[179] and learn about local Community Supported Agriculture (CSA)[180] programs in your area.

For a list of fish and their mercury levels, go to NRDC's wallet guide at www.nrdc.org.[181]

For a list of foods that are high in pesticide residues, visit the Environmental Working Group's "dirty dozen" list at www.ewg.org/foodnews/dirty-dozen.php.[182] When possible, choose organic versions of these foods.

To learn more about toxic skincare ingredients, visit the Environmental Working Group's Skin Deep database at www.ewg.org/skindeep.[183]

To find a naturopathic doctor in your area, visit the American Association of Physicians website at www.naturopathic.org[184] or the Institute for Natural Medicine at www.naturemed.org/find-an-nd.[185]

To find a functional medicine practitioner in your area, visit the Institute for Functional Medicine at www.ifm.org/find-a-practitioner/.[186]

ACKNOWLEDGMENTS

There are so many people to whom I'd love to express gratitude for their support of this book, and they include:

My colleagues who joined me for the "Sister Summers Solstice" gathering for a weekend of reconnecting and interviews for the *Hormones, Health, and Harmony* docuseries. You'll see pictures of some of these women throughout this book.

Dr. Hyla Cass for the feedback on chapter 3 ("Mood and Memory") as one of the leading integrative psychiatrists in the country. You can find a beautiful photo of her on page 11.

Rachael Pontillo for her creative support on the DIY skincare recipes in this book.

The Spa Dr. Team, especially Linda Higgins and Katie Jackson, who helped lighten my load while I was writing this book and ensuring The Spa Dr. continues to have the best customer support of any online skincare company.

My husband, Barclay Burns, for his loving support and encouragement.

My three children, Tiernan, Truan, and Thalia, for continuing to be my biggest teachers in life. I love you to the moon and back!

My family full of powerful women leaders—my mother, Gwen; my two aunts, Linda and Karen; and my two older sisters, Ayn and Challen, for all the life lessons growing up and their continued inspiration as strong and creative women.

My father, Bill, who passed away several years ago but whose appreciation for nature planted a seed in me years ago that has been the main driver of my work.

For the Navajo people in Monument Valley and other Native Americans who remind me of our connection to Mother Earth.

For my spiritual journey and learning to trust and lean into Divine Guidance.

NOTES

1   "beauty," Merriam-Webster, https://www.merriam-webster.com/dictionary/beauty.

2   "Depression on the Rise During COVID-19: Resources for Patients and Their Families," Massachusetts General Hospital News, June 25, 2020, https://www.massgeneral.org/news/coronavirus/depression-on-rise-during-covid-19.

3   Paul R. Albert, "Why is depression more prevalent in women?" *Journal of Psychiatry & Neuroscience* 40, no. 4 (2015): 219–21, doi:10.1503/jpn.150205.

4   "Who We Are," Endocrine Society About Us Page, https://www.endocrine.org/about-us.

5   Trevor Cates, "How Your Thyroid Reacts to Skin Care Ingredients," The Spa Dr., https://thespadr.com/thyroid-harmful-skin-care-ingredients/.

6   Åshild Bjørnerem, Bjørn Straume, Pål Øian et al., "Seasonal Variation of Estradiol, Follicle Stimulating Hormone, and Dehydroepiandrosterone Sulfate in Women and Men," *The Journal of Clinical Endocrinology & Metabolism* 91, no. 10 (2006): 3798–802, doi:10.1210/jc.2006-0866.

7   Michael R. McClung, "The relationship between bone mineral density and fracture risk," *Current Osteoporosis Reports* 3, no. 2 (2005): 57–63, doi:10.1007/s11914-005-0005-y.

8   Daniele Santi, Giorgia Spaggiari, Giulia Brigante et al., "Semi-annual seasonal pattern of serum thyrotropin in adults," *Scientific Reports* 9 (2019), doi:10.1038/s41598-019-47349-4.

9   Trevor Cates, "The Scary Facts about Sugar and Your Skin," The Spa Dr., https://thespadr.com/the-scary-facts-about-sugar-and-your-skin/.

10 Roger Persson, Anne Helene Garde, Ase Marie Hansen et al., "Seasonal variation in human salivary cortisol concentration," *Chronobiology International* 25, no. 6 (2008): 923–37, doi:10.1080/07420520802553648.

11 Lars Berglund, Christian Berne, Kurt Svärdsudd et al., "Seasonal variations of insulin sensitivity from a euglycemic insulin clamp in elderly men," *Upsala Journal of Medical Sciences* 117, no. 1 (2012): 35–40, doi:10.3109/03009734.2011.628422.

12 Adam G. Tabák, Christian Herder, Wolfgang Rathmann et al., "Prediabetes: A high-risk state for developing diabetes," *Lancet* 379 (2012): 2279–90, doi:10.1016/S0140-6736(12)60283-9.

13 Xiaoying Xu, Xiaoyan Liu, Shuran Ma et al., "Association of Melatonin Production with Seasonal Changes, Low Temperature, and Immuno-Responses in Hamsters," *Molecules* 23, no. 3 (2018): 703, doi:10.3390/molecules23030703.

14 Xiaoying Xu, Xiaoyan Liu, Shuran Ma et al., "Association of Melatonin Production with Seasonal Changes, Low Temperature, and Immuno-Responses in Hamsters," *Molecules* 23, no. 3 (2018): 703, doi:10.3390/molecules23030703.

15 Azade Shabani, Fatemeh Foroozanfard, Elham Kavossian et al., "Effects of melatonin administration on mental health parameters, metabolic and genetic profiles in women with polycystic ovary syndrome: a randomized, double-blind, placebo-controlled trial," *Journal of Affective Disorders* 250 (2019): 51–56, doi:10.1016/j.jad.2019.02.066.

16 James M. Olcese, "Melatonin and Female Reproduction: An Expanding Universe," *Frontiers in Endocrinology* 11 (2020): 85, doi:10.3389/fendo.2020.00085.

17 Gail A. Greendale, Paula Witt-Enderby, Arun S. Karlamangla et al., "Melatonin Patterns and Levels During the Human Menstrual Cycle and After Menopause," *Journal of the Endocrine Society* 4, no. 11 (2020), doi:10.1210/jendso/bvaa115.

18 S. Epperlein, C. Gebhardt, K. Rohde et al., "The Effect of FGF21 and Its Genetic Variants on Food and Drug Cravings, Adipokines and Metabolic Traits," Biomedicines. U.S. National Library of Medicine. Accessed February 3, 2022. https://pubmed.ncbi.nlm.nih.gov/33805553/.

19 Shaina Cahill, Erin Tuplin, and Matthew R. Holahan, "Circannual changes in stress and feeding hormones and their effect on food-seeking behaviors," *Frontiers in Neuroscience* 7 (2013): 140, doi:10.3389/fnins.2013.00140.

20 K. Uvnäs-Moberg, "Oxytocin linked antistress effects—the relaxation and growth response," *Acta Physiologica Scandinavica, Supplementum* 640 (1997): 38–42, https://pubmed.ncbi.nlm.nih.gov/9401603/.

21 Heidi H. Kong and Julia A. Segre, "Skin Microbiome: Looking Back to Move Forward," *Journal of Investigative Dermatology* 132, no. 3 (2012): 933–39, doi:10.1038/jid.2011.417.

22 Iman Salem, Amy Ramser, Nancy Isham et al., "The Gut Microbiome as a Major Regulator of the Gut-Skin Axis," *Frontiers in Microbiology* 9 (2018): 1459, doi:10.3389/fmicb.2018.01459.

23 Iman Salem, Amy Ramser, Nancy Isham et al., "The Gut Microbiome as a Major Regulator of the Gut-Skin Axis," *Frontiers in Microbiology* 9 (2018): 1459, doi:10.3389/fmicb.2018.01459.

24 H. Hambers, S. Piessens, A. Bloem, et al., "Natural skin surface pH is on average below 5, which is beneficial for its resident flora," *International Journal of Cosmetic Science* 28, no. 5 (2006): 359–70, doi:10.1111/j.1467-2494.2006.00344.x.

25 Y. C. Jung, E. J. Kim, J. C. Cho et al., "Effect of skin pH for wrinkle formation on Asian: Korean, Vietnamese and Singaporean," *Journal of the European Academy of Dermatology and Venereology* 27, no. 3 (2012): 328–32, doi:10.1111/j.1468-3083.2012.04660.x.

26 E. G. Lopes, D. A. Moreira, P. Gullón et al., "Topical application of probiotics in skin: adhesion, antimicrobial and antibiofilm *in vitro* assays," *Journal of Applied Microbiology* 122, no. 2 (2016): 450–61, doi:10.1111/jam.13349.

27 F. H. Al-Ghazzewi and R. F. Tester, "Impact of prebiotics and probiotics on skin health," *Beneficial Microbes* 5, no. 2 (2014): 99–107, doi:10.3920/BM2013.0040.

28 L-C Lew and M-T Liong, "Bioactives from probiotics for dermal health: functions and benefits," *Journal of Applied Microbiology* 114, no. 5 (2013): 1241–53, doi:10.1111/jam.12137.

29 David H. Martin, "The Microbiota of the Vagina and Its Influence on Women's Health and Disease," *American Journal of the Medical Sciences* 343, no. 1 (2012): 2–9, doi:10.1097/MAJ.0b013e31823ea228.

30 Felicia M. T. Lewis, Kyle T. Bernstein, and Sevgi O. Aral, "Vaginal Microbiome and Its Relationship to Behavior, Sexual Health, and Sexually Transmitted Diseases," *Obstetrics & Gynecology* 129, no. 4 (2017): 643–54, doi:10.1097/AOG.0000000000001932.

31 Jessica Maiuolo, Micaela Gliozzi, Vincenzo Musolino et al., "The Contribution of Gut Microbiota–Brain Axis in the Development of Brain Disorders," *Frontiers in Neuroscience* 15 (2021), doi:10.3389/fnins.2021.616883.

32 N. C. Wiley, J. F. Cryan, T. G. Dinan et al., "Production of Psychoactive Metabolites by Gut Bacteria," *Microbes and the Mind: The Impact of the Microbiome on Mental Health* 32 (2021): 74–99, doi:10.1159/000510419.

33 Aitak Farzi, Esther E. Fröhlich, and Peter Holzer, "Gut Microbiota and the Neuroendocrine System," *Neurotherapeutics* 15, no. 1 (2018): 5–22, doi:10.1007/s13311-017-0600-5.

34 Aitak Farzi, Esther E. Fröhlich, and Peter Holzer, "Gut Microbiota and the Neuroendocrine System," *Neurotherapeutics* 15, no. 1 (2018): 5–22, doi:10.1007/s13311-017-0600-5.

35 "Gamma-Aminobutyric Acid," ScienceDirect, https://www.sciencedirect.com/topics/medicine-and-dentistry/gamma-aminobutyric-acid.

36 D. D. Murphy, N. B. Cole, V. Greenberger et al., "Estradiol increases dendritic spine density by reducing GABA neurotransmission in hippocampal neurons," *Journal of Neuroscience* 18, no. 7 (1998): 2550–9, doi:10.1523/JNEUROSCI.18-07-02550.1998.

37 G. A. van Wingen, F. van Broekhoven, R. J. Verkes et al., "Progesterone selectively increases amygdala reactivity in women," *Molecular Psychiatry* 13, no. 3 (2008): 325–33, doi:10.1038/sj.mp.4002030.

38 Evert Boonstra, Roy de Kleijn, Lorenza S. Colzato et al., "Neurotransmitters as food supplements: the effects of GABA on brain and behavior," *Frontiers in Psychology* 6 (2015), doi:10.3389/fpsyg.2015.01520.

39 Behnood Abbasi, Masud Kimiagar, Khosro Sadeghniiat et al., "The effect of magnesium supplementation on primary insomnia in elderly: A double-blind placebo-controlled clinical trial," *Journal of Research in Medical Sciences* 17, no. 12 (2012): 1161–9, https://pubmed.ncbi.nlm.nih.gov/23853635/.

40 Chris C. Streeter, Patricia L. Gerbarg, Richard P. Brown et al., "Thalamic Gamma Aminobutyric Acid Level Changes in Major Depressive Disorder After a 12-Week Iyengar Yoga and Coherent Breathing Intervention," *The Journal of Alternative and Complementary Medicine* 26, no. 3 (2020), doi:10.1089/acm.2019.0234.

41 Simon N. Young, "How to increase serotonin in the human brain without drugs," *Journal of Psychiatry & Neuroscience* 32, no. 6 (2007): 394–99, https://www.ncbi.nlm.nih.gov/pmc/articles/PMC2077351/.

42 Brigham and Women's Hospital, "Anxiety linked to shortened telomeres, accelerated aging," ScienceDaily, July 11, 2012, https://www.sciencedaily.com/releases/2012/07/120711210102.htm.

43 Nicola S. Schutte and John M. Malouff, "A meta-analytic review of the effects of mindfulness meditation on telomerase activity," *Psychoneuroendocrinology* 42 (2014): 45–48, doi:10.1016/j.psyneuen.2013.12.017.

44 Raphaëlle Chaix, Maria Jesús Alvarez-López, Maud Fagny et al., "Epigenetic clock analysis in long-term meditators," *Psychoneuroendocrinology* 85 (2017): 210–14, doi:10.1016.j.psyneuen.2017.08.016.

45 Hayley Robinson, Paul Jarrett, and Elizabeth Broadbent, "The Effects of Relaxation Before or After Skin Damage on Skin Barrier Recovery: A Preliminary Study," *Psychosomatic Medicine* 77, no. 8 (2015): 844–52, doi:10.1097/PSY.0000000000000222.

46 Jim Robbins, "How immersing yourself in nature benefits your health," *PBS NewsHour*, January 13, 2020, https://www.pbs.org/newshour/health/how-immersing-yourself-in-nature-benefits-your-health.

47 Marvin G. Knittel, "Could the Seasons Affect Your Mood?" *Psychology Today*, June 12, 2017, https://www.psychologytoday.com/us/blog/how-help-friend/201706/could-the-seasons-affect-your-mood-1.

48 Asher Y. Rosinger, Anne-Marie Chang, Orfeu M. Buxton et al., "Short sleep duration is associated with inadequate hydration: cross-cultural evidence from US and Chinese adults," *Sleep* 42, no. 2 (2019), doi:10.1093/sleep/zsy210.

49 Richard G. Stevens, "Light-at-night, circadian disruption and breast cancer: assessment of existing evidence," *International Journal of Epidemiology* 38, no. 4 (2009): 963–70, doi:10.1093/ije/dyp178.

50 T. A. Bedrosian, R. J. Nelson, "Influence of the modern light environment on mood," *Molecular Psychiatry* 18, no. 7 (2013): 751–7, doi:10.1038/mp.2013.70.

51 Laura K. Fonken, Joanna L. Workman, James C. Walton et al., "Light at night increases body mass by shifting the time of food intake," *PNAS* 107, no. 43 (2010): 18,664–9, doi:10.1073/pnas.1008734107.

52 Ari Shechter, Elijah Wookhyun Kim, Marie-Pierre St-Onge et al., "Blocking nocturnal blue light for insomnia: A randomized controlled trial," *Journal of Psychiatric Research* 96 (2018): 196–202, doi:10.1016/j.jpsychires.2017.10.015.

53 Kazue Okamoto-Mizuno and Koh Mizuno, "Effects of thermal environment on sleep and circadian rhythm," *Journal of Physiological Anthropology* 31 (2012), doi:10.1186/1880-6805-31-14.

54 Danielle Pacheco, "The Best Temperature for Sleep," Sleep Foundation, June 24, 2021, https://www.sleepfoundation.org/bedroom-environment/best-temperature-for-sleep.

55 Marc A. Russo, Danielle M. Santarelli, and Dean O'Rourke, "The physiological effects of slow breathing in the healthy human," *Breathe* 13, no. 4 (2017): 298–309, doi:10.1183/20734735.009817.

56 Shaina Cahill, Erin Tuplin, and Matthew R. Holahan, "Circannual changes in stress and feeding hormones and their effect on food-seeking behaviors," *Frontiers in Neuroscience* 7 (2013): 140, doi:10.3389/fnins.2013.00140.

57 Shaina Cahill, Erin Tuplin, and Matthew R. Holahan, "Circannual changes in stress and feeding hormones and their effect on food-seeking behaviors," *Frontiers in Neuroscience* 7 (2013): 140, doi:10.3389/fnins.2013.00140.

58 Avichai Tendler, Alon Bar, Netta Mendelsohn-Cohen et al., "Hormone seasonality in medical records suggests circannual endocrine circuits," *PNAS* 118 (2021), doi:10.1073/pnas.2003926118.

59 A. Kauppila, A. Pakarinen, P. Kirkinen et al., "The effect of season on the circulating concentrations of anterior pituitary, ovarian and adrenal cortex hormones and hormone binding proteins in the subarctic area; evidence of increased activity of the pituitary-ovarian axis in spring," *Gynecological Endocrinology* 1, no. 2 (1987): 137–50, doi:10.3109/09513598709030678.

60 Zuying Chen, Linda Godfrey-Bailey, Isaac Schiff et al., "Impact of seasonal variation, age and smoking status on human semen parameters: The Massachusetts General Hospital experience," *Journal of Experimental & Clinical Assisted Reproduction* 1 (2004): 2, doi:10.1186/1743-1050-1-2.

61 Shahla M. Wunderlich, Charles Feldman, Shannon Kane et al., "Nutritional quality of organic, conventional, and seasonally grown broccoli using vitamin C as a marker," *International Journal of Food Sciences and Nutrition* 59, no 1 (2008): 34–45, doi:10.1080/09637480701453637.

62 Marica Krajcovicová-Kudláčková, Martina Valachovicová, and Pavel Blazícek, "Seasonal folate serum concentrations at different nutrition," *CEJPH* 21, no. 1 (2013): 36–8, doi:10.21101/cejph.a3785.

63 Winfried E. H. Blum, Sophie Zechmeister-Boltenstern, and Katharina M. Keiblinger, "Does Soil Contribute to the Human Gut Microbiome?" *Microorganisms* 7, no. 9 (2019): 287, doi:10.3390/microorganisms7090287.

64 James M. MacDonald, "Demand, Information, and Competition: Why Do Food Prices Fall at Seasonal Demand Peaks?" *Journal of Industrial Economics* 48, no. 1 (2003): 27–45, doi:10.1111/1467-6451.00111.

65 P. V. Mahajan, O. J. Caleb, Z. Singh et al., "Postharvest treatments of fresh produce," *Philosophical Transactions: Mathematical, Physical and Engineering Sciences*, 372 (2017), doi:10.1098/rsta.2013.0309.

66 Gianfranco Romanazzi, Erica Feliziani, Silvia Bautista Baños et al., "Shelf life extension of fresh fruit and vegetables by chitosan treatment," *Critical Reviews in Food Science and Nutrition* 57, no. 3 (2017): 579–601, doi:10.1080/10408398.2014.900474.

67 J. Webb, Adrian G. Williams, Emma Hope et al., "Do foods imported into the UK have a greater environmental impact than the same foods produced within the UK?" *International Journal of Life Cycle Assessment* 18 (2013): 132,543, doi:10.1007/s11367-013-0576-2.

68 A. Mancini, R. Festa, V. Di Donna et al., "Hormones and antioxidant systems: role of pituitary and pituitary-dependent axes," *Journal of Endocrinological Investigation* 33, no. 6 (2010): 422–33, doi:10.1007/BF03346615.

69 Bartley G. Hoebel, Nicole M. Avena, Miriam E. Bocarsly et al., "A Behavioral and Circuit Model Based on Sugar Addiction in Rats," *Journal of Addiction Medicine* 3, no. 1 (2009): 3341, doi:10.1097/ADM.0b013e31819aa621.

70 Sam Escobar, "The Number of Makeup Products the Average Woman Owns Is Just Plain Shocking," *Good Housekeeping*, October 14, 2015, https://www.goodhousekeeping.com/beauty/makeup/a34976/average-makeup-products-owned/.

71 "Personal Care Products Safety Act Would Improve Cosmetics Safety," Environmental Working Group, https://www.ewg.org/personal-care-products-safety-act-would-improve-cosmetics-safety.

72 "Prohibited & Restricted Ingredients in Cosmetics," FDA, last updated August 24, 2020, https://www.fda.gov/cosmetics/cosmetics-laws-regulations/prohibited-restricted-ingredients-cosmetics#prohibited.

73 Erika S. Koeppe, Kelly K. Ferguson, Justin A. Colacino et al., "Relationship between urinary triclosan and paraben concentrations and serum thyroid measures in NHANES 2007–2008," *Science of The Total Environment* 445–446 (2013): 299–305, doi:10.1016/j.scitotenv.2012.12.052.

74 Manori J. Silva, Dana B. Barr, John A. Reidy et al., "Urinary levels of seven phthalate metabolites in the U.S. population from the National Health and Nutrition Examination Survey (NHANES) 1999–2000," *Environmental Health Perspectives* 112, no. 3 (2004): 331–8, doi:10.1289/ehp.6723.

75 Douglas A. Haines, Gurusankar Saravanabhavan, Kate Werry et al., "An overview of human biomonitoring of environmental chemicals in the Canadian Health Measures Survey: 2007–2019," *International Journal of Hygiene and Environmental Health* 220, no. 2 (2017): 13–28, doi:10.1016/j.ijheh.2016.08.002.

76 Murali K. Matta, Jeffry Florian, Robbert Zusterzeel et al., "Effect of Sunscreen Application on Plasma Concentration of Sunscreen Active Ingredients: A Randomized Clinical Trial," *JAMA* 323, no. 3 (2020): 256–267, doi:10.1001/jama.2019.20747.

77 "Lead in food: A hidden health threat," Environmental Defense Fund, June 14, 2017, https://www.edf.org/health/lead-food-hidden-health-threat.

78 "Learn about Lead," United States Environmental Protection Agency, https://www.epa.gov/lead/learn-about-lead.

79 "What to do about mercury in fish," Harvard Health Publishing, July 28, 2017, https://www.health.harvard.edu/staying-healthy/what-to-do-about-mercury-in-fish.

80 "PCBs in fish and shellfish," EDF Seafood Selector, https://seafood.edf.org/pcbs-fish-and-shellfish.

81 J. Rhee, T. M. Vance, R. Lim et al., "Association of blood mercury levels with nonmelanoma skin cancer in the U.S.A. using National Health and Nutrition Examination Survey data (2003–2016)," *British Journal of Dermatology* 183, no. 3 (2020): 480–7, doi:10.1111/bjd.18797.

82 Beverly S. Rubin, "Bisphenol A: an endocrine disruptor with widespread exposure and multiple effects," *Journal of Steroid Biochemistry and Molecular Biology* 127 (2011): 27–34, doi:10.1016/j.jsbmb.2011.05.002.

83 Raquel Moral, Richard Wang, Irma H. Russo et al., "Effect of prenatal exposure to the endocrine disruptor bisphenol A on mammary gland morphology and gene expression signature," *Journal of Endocrinology* 196, no. 1 (2008): 101–12, doi:10.1667/JOE-07-0056.

84 Anoop Shankar and Srinivas Teppala, "Relationship between urinary bisphenol A levels and diabetes mellitus," *Journal of Clinical Endocrinology & Metabolism* 96, no. 12 (2011): 3822–6, doi:10.1210/jc.2011-1682.

85 Eleni Kandaraki, Antonis Chatzigeorgiou, Sarantis Livadas et al., "Endocrine disruptors and polycystic ovary syndrome (PCOS): elevated serum levels of bisphenol A in women with PCOS," *Journal of Clinical Endocrinology & Metabolism* 96, no. 3 (2011), doi:10.1210/jc.2010-1658.

86 E. Mok-lin, S. Ehrlich, P. L. Williams et al., "Urinary bisphenol A concentrations and ovarian response among women undergoing IVF," *International Journal of Andrology* 33, no. 2 (2010): 385–93, doi:10.111/j.1365-2605.2009.01014.x.

87 Elliyana Nadia Hamidi, Parvaneh Hajeg, Jinap Selamat et al., "Polycyclic Aromatic Hydrocarbons (PAHs) and Their Bioaccessibility in Meat: a Tool for Assessing Human Cancer Risk," *Asian Pacific Journal of Cancer Prevention* 17, no. 1 (2016): 15–23, doi:10.7314/apjcp.2016.17.1.15.

88 S. Seely and D. F. Horrobin, "Diet and breast cancer: the possible connection with sugar consumption," *Medical Hypotheses* 11, no. 3 (1983): 319–27, doi:10.1016/0306-9877(83)90095-6.

89 James J. DiNicolantonio, James H. O'Keefe, and Sean C. Lucan, "Added fructose: a principal driver of type 2 diabetes mellitus and its consequences," *Mayo Clinic Proceedings* 90, no. 3 (2015): 372–81, doi:10.1016/j.mayocp.2014.12.019.

90 Kimber L. Stanhope and Peter J. Havel, "Fructose consumption: considerations for future research on its effects on adipose distribution, lipid metabolism, and insulin sensitivity in humans," *Journal of Nutrition* 139, no. 6 (2009), doi:10.3945/jn.109.106641.

91 R. M. Bostick, J. D. Potter, L. H. Kushi et al., "Sugar, meat, and fat intake, and non-dietary risk factors for colon cancer incidence in Iowa women (United States)," *Cancer Causes & Control* 5, no. 1 (1994): 38–52, doi:10.1007/BF01830725.

92 Kimber L. Stanhope, Jean-Marc Schwarz, and Peter J. Havel, "Adverse metabolic effects of dietary fructose: results from the recent epidemiological, clinical, and mechanistic studies," *Current Opinion in Lipidology* 24, no. 3 (2013): 198–206, doi:10.1097/MOL.0b013e3283613bca.

93 "Dirty Dozen: EWG's 2021 Shopper's Guide to Pesticides in Produce," Environmental Working Group, https://www.ewg.org/foodnews/dirty-dozen.php.

94 "Mercury in Fish: A Guide to Protecting Your Family's Health," Natural Resources Defense Council, https://www.nrdc.org/sites/default/files/walletcard.pdf.

95 Virginia Boccardi, Giuseppe Paolisso, and Patrizia Mecocci, "Nutrition and lifestyle in healthy aging: the telomerase challenge," *Aging* 8, no. 1 (2016): 12–15, doi:10.18632/aging.100886.

96 Dennis T. Villareal, Luigi Fontana, Sai Krupa Das et al., "Effect of Two-Year Caloric Restriction on Bone Metabolism and Bone Mineral Density in Non-obese Younger Adults: a Randomized Clinical Trial," *Journal of Bone and Mineral Research* 31, no. 1 (2016): 40–51, doi:10.1002/jbmr.2701.

97 Stephen J. Genuis, Sanjay Beesoon, Rebecca A. Lobo et al., "Human Elimination of Phthalate Compounds: Blood, Urine, and Sweat (BUS) Study," *Scientific World Journal* (2012), doi:10.1100/2012/615068.

98 Madhuri Tolahunase, Rajesh Sagar, and Rima Dada, "Impact of Yoga and Meditation on Cellular Aging in Apparently Healthy Individuals: A Prospective, Open-Label Single-Arm Exploratory Study," *Oxidative Medicine and Cellular Longevity* (2017), doi:10.1155/2017/7928981.

99 Ying Chen and John Lyga, "Brain-Skin Connection: Stress, Inflammation and Skin Aging," *Inflammation & Allergy Drug Targets* 13, no. 3 (2014): 177–90, doi:10.2174/18715281136661400522104422.

100 Petra Clara Arck, Bori Handjiski, Eva M. J. Peters et al., "Topical minoxidil counteracts stress-induced hair growth inhibition in mice," *Experimental Dermatology* 12, no. 5 (2003): 580–90, doi:10.1034/j.1600-0625.2003.00028.

101 Michael A. Bachelor and G. Tim Bowden, "UVA-mediated activation of signaling pathways involved in skin tumor promotion and progression," *Seminars in Cancer Biology* 14, no. 2 (2004): 131–38, doi:10.1016/j.semcancer.2003.09.017.

102 Daniele Santi, Giorgia Spaggiari, Giulia Brigante et al., "Semi-annual seasonal pattern of serum thyrotropin in adults," *Scientific Reports* 9 (2019), doi:10.1038/s41598-019-47349-4.

103 Rathish Nair and Arun Maseeh, "Vitamin D: The 'sunshine' vitamin," *Journal of Pharmacology & Pharmacotherapeutics* 3, no. 2 (2012): 118–26, doi:10.4103/0976-500X.95506.

104 Laura M. Hall, Michael G. Kimlin, Pavel A. Aronov et al., "Vitamin D intake needed to maintain target serum 25-hydroxyvitamin D concentrations in participants with low sun exposure and dark skin pigmentation is substantially higher than current recommendations," *Journal of Nutrition* 140, no. 3 (2010): 542–50, doi:10.3945/jn.109.115253.

105 James M. Olcese, "Melatonin and Female Reproduction: An Expanding Universe," *Frontiers in Endocrinology* 11 (2020): 85, doi:10.3389/fendo.2020.00085.

106 Laura R. LaChance and Drew Ramsey, "Antidepressant foods: An evidence-based nutrient profiling system for depression," *World Journal of Psychiatry* 8, no. 3 (2018): 97–104, doi:10.5498/wjp.v8.i3.97.

107 Camille Lassale, G. David Batty, Amaria Baghdadli et al., "Healthy dietary indices and risk of depressive outcomes: a systematic review and meta-analysis of observational studies," *Molecular Psychiatry* 24, no. 7 (2019): 965–96, doi:10.1038/s41380-018-0237-8.

108 Qurrat-ul-Aen Inam, Huma Ikram, Erum Shireen et al., "Effects of sugar rich diet on brain serotonin, hyperphagia and anxiety in animal model of both genders," *Pakistan Journal of Pharmaceutical Sciences* 29, no. 3 (2016): 757–63, https://pubmed.ncbi.nlm.nih.gov/27166525/.

109 Sammi R. Chekroud, Ralitza Gueorguieva, Amanda B. Zheutlin et al., "Association between physical exercise and mental health in 1.2 million individuals in the USA between 2011 and 2015: a cross-sectional study," *Lancet Psychiatry* 5, no. 9 (2018): 739–46, doi:10.1016/S2215-0366(18)30227-X.

110 Sari M. van Anders, Elizabeth Hampson, and Neil V. Watson, "Seasonality, waist-to-hip ratio, and salivary testosterone," *Psychoneuroendocrinology* 31, no. 7 (2006): 895–9, doi:10.1016/j.psyneuen.2006.03.002.

111 Gregory N. Bratman, J. Paul Hamilton, Kevin S. Hahn et al., "Nature experience reduces rumination and subgenual prefrontal cortex activation," *PNAS* 112 (2015): 8567–72, doi:10.1073/pnas.1510459112.

112 Jim Robbins, "How immersing yourself in nature benefits your health," *PBS NewsHour*, January 13, 2020, https://www.pbs.org/newshour/health/how-immersing-yourself-in-nature-benefits-your-health.

113 Karen A. Baikie and Kay Wilhelm, "Emotional and physical health benefits of expressive writing," *Advances in Psychiatric Treatment* 11 (2005): 338–46, doi:10.1192/apt.11.5.338.

114 E. Mohandas, "Neurobiology of Spirituality," *Mens Sana Monographs* 6, no. 1 (2008): 63–80, doi:10.4103/0973-1229.33001.

115 Mariana G. Figueiro, Bryan Steverson, Judith Heerwagen et al., "The impact of daytime light exposures on sleep and mood in office workers," *Sleep Health* 3, no. 3 (2017): 204–15, doi:10.1016/j.sleh.2017.03.005.

116 Veronika Pechová and Jan Gajdziok, "Possibilities of using sodium hyaluronate in pharmaceutical and medical fields," *Ceská a Slovenská Farmacie* 66, no. 4 (2017): 154–9, https://pubmed.ncbi.nlm.nih.gov/29351375/.

117 Marya S. Sabir, Mark R. Haussler, Sanchita Mallick et al., "Optimal vitamin D spurs serotonin: 1,25-dihydroxyvitamin D represses serotonin reuptake transport (*SERT*) and degradation (*MAO-A*) gene expression in cultured rat serotonergic neuronal cell lines," *Genes & Nutrition* 13 (2018): 19, doi:10.1186/s12263-018-0605-7.

118 Daniele Santi, Giorgia Spaggiari, Giulia Brigante et al., "Semi-annual seasonal pattern of serum thyrotropin in adults," *Scientific Reports* 9 (2019), doi:10.1038/s41598-019-47349-4.

119 Marica Krajcovicová-Kudláčková, Martina Valachovicová, and Pavel Blazícek, "Seasonal folate serum concentrations at different nutrition," *CEJPH* 21, no. 1 (2013): 36–8, doi:10.21101/cejph.a3785.

120 Prashanthi Vemuri, Timothy G. Lesnick, Scott A. Przybelski et al., "Association of Lifetime Intellectual Enrichment with Cognitive Decline in the Older Population," *JAMA Neurol.* 71, no. 8 (2014): 1017–24, doi:10.1001/jamaneurol.2014.963.

121 Randy A. Sansone and Lori A. Sansone, "Sunshine, Serotonin, and Skin: A Partial Explanation for Seasonal Patterns in Psychopathology?" *Innovations in Clinical Neuroscience* 10 (2013): 20–24, https://www.ncbi.nlm.nih.gov/pmc/articles/PMC3779905/.

122 Thilo Gambichler, Armin Bader, Mirjana Vojvodic et al., "Impact of UVA exposure on psychological parameters and circulating serotonin and melatonin," *BMC Dermatology* 2 (2002): 6, doi:10.1186/1471-5945-2-6.

123 Kimberley J. Smith, Shannon Gavey, Natalie E. Riddell et al., "The association between loneliness, social isolation and inflammation: A systematic review and meta-analysis," *Neuroscience & Biobehavioral Reviews* 112 (2020): 519–41, doi:10.1016/j.neubiorev.2020.02.002.

124 Moriel Zelikowsky, May Hui, Tomomi Karigo et al., "The Neuropeptide Tac2 Controls a Distributed Brain State Induced by Chronic Social Isolation Stress," *Cell* 173, no 5 (2018): 1265-79, doi:10.1016/j.cell.2018.03.037.

125 JongEun Yim, "Therapeutic Benefits of Laughter in Mental Health: A Theoretical Review," *Tohoku Journal of Experimental Medicine* 239, no. 3 (2016): 243–9, doi:10.1620/tjem.239.243.

126 R. I. M. Dunbar, Anna Frangou, Felix Grainger et al., "Laughter influences social bonding but not prosocial generosity to friends and strangers," *PLoS One* 16, no 8 (2021), doi:10.1371/journal.pone.0256229.

127 Adrián Pérez-Aranda, Jennifer Hofmann, Albert Feliu-Soler et al., "Laughing away the pain: A narrative review of humour, sense of humour and pain," *European Journal of Pain* 23, no. 2 (2019): 220–33, doi:10.1002/ejp.1309.

128 Dae Hun Kim, Young Jin Je, Chang Deok Kim et al., "Can Platelet-rich Plasma Be Used for Skin Rejuvenation? Evaluation of Effects of Platelet-rich Plasma on Human Derman Fibroblast," *Annals of Dermatology* 23, no. 4 (2011): 424–31, doi:10.5021/ad.2011.23.4.424.

129 Jim Robbins, "How immersing yourself in nature benefits your health," *PBS NewsHour*, January 13, 2020, https://www.pbs.org/newshour/health/how-immersing-yourself-in-nature-benefits-your-health.

130 Winfried E. H. Blum, Sophie Zechmeister-Boltenstern, and Katharina M. Keiblinger, "Does Soil Contribute to the Human Gut Microbiome?" *Microorganisms* 7, no. 9 (2019): 287, doi:10.3390/microorganisms7090287.

131 B. C. Nindl, W. J. Kraemer, L. A. Gotshalk et al., "Testosterone responses after resistance exercise in women: influence of regional fat distribution," *International Journal of Sport Nutrition and Exercise Metabolism* 11, no. 4 (2001): 451–65, doi:10.1123/ijsnem.11.4.451.

132 Richard J. Godfrey, Zahra Madgwick, and Gregory P. Whyte, "The exercise-induced growth hormone response in athletes," *Sports Medicine* 33, no. 8 (2003): 599–613, doi:10.2165/00007256-200333080-00005.

133 E. E. Hill, E. Zac, C. Battaglini et al., "Exercise and circulating cortisol levels: the intensity threshold effect," *Journal of Endocrinological Investigation* 31, no. 7 (2008): 587–91, doi:10.1007/BF03345606.

134 Diana Crisan, Iulia Roman, Maria Crisan et al., "The role of vitamin C in pushing back the boundaries of skin aging: an ultrasonographic approach," *Clinical, Cosmetic and Investigational Dermatology* 8 (2015): 463–70, dio:10.2147/CCID.S84903.

135 Konstantin V. Danilenko, Oksana Y. Sergceva, and Evgeniy G. Verevkin, "Menstrual cycles are influenced by sunshine," *Gynecological Endocrinology* 27, no. 9 (2011): 711–16, doi:10.3109/09513590.2010.521266.

136 Åshild Bjørnerem, Bjørn Straume, Pål Øian et al., "Seasonal Variation of Estradiol, Follicle Stimulating Hormone, and Dehydroepiandrosterone Sulfate in Women and Men," *The Journal of Clinical Endocrinology & Metabolism* 91, no. 10 (2006): 3798–802, doi:10.1210/jc.2006-0866.

137 Randy A. Sansone and Lori A. Sansone, "Sunshine, Serotonin, and Skin: A Partial Explanation for Seasonal Patterns in Psychopathology?" *Innovations in Clinical Neuroscience* 10 (2013): 20–24, https://www.ncbi.nlm.nih.gov/pmc/articles/PMC3779905/.

138 L. Y. Matsuoka, L. Ide, J. Wortsman et al., "Sunscreens suppress cutaneous vitamin D_3 synthesis," *Journal of Clinical Endocrinology & Metabolism* 64, no. 6 (1987): 1165–8, doi:10.1210/jcem-64-6-1165.

139 Jee-Hye Yoo, "The psychological effects of water-based exercise in older adults: An integrative review," *Geriatric Nursing* 41, no. 6 (2020): 717–23, doi:10.1016/j.gerinurse.2020.04.019.

140 Chris Callewaert, Prawira Hutapea, Tom Van de Wiele et al., "Deodorants and antiperspirants affect the axillary bacterial community," *Archives of Dermatological Research* 306, no. 8 (2014): 701–10, doi:10.1007/s00403-014-1487-1.

141 Lara S. Franco, Danielle F. Shanahan, and Richard A. Fuller, "A Review of the Benefits of Nature Experiences: More Than Meets the Eye," *International Journal of Environmental Research and Public Health* 14, no. 8 (2017): 864, doi:10.3390/ijerph14080864.

142 Howard Frumkin, Gregory N. Bratman, Sara Jo Breslow et al., "Nature Contact and Human Health: A Research Agenda," *Environmental Health Perspectives* 125, no. 7 (2017), doi:10.1289/EHP1663.

143 Theoharis C. Theoharides and Leonard Bielory, "Mast cells and mast cell mediators as targets of dietary supplements," *Annals of Allergy, Asthma & Immunology* 93 (2004), doi:10.1016/s1081-1206(10)61484-6.

144 Andrzej T. Slominski, Michal A. Zmijewski, Igor Semak et al., "Melatonin, mitochondria, and the skin," *Cellular and Molecular Life Sciences* 74 (2017): 3913–25, doi:10.1007/s00018-017-2617-7.

145 Ibrar Anjum, Syeda S. Jaffery, Muniba Fayyaz et al., "The Role of Vitamin D in Brain Health: A Mini Literature Review," *Cureus* 10, no. 7 (2018), doi:10.7759/cureus.2960.

146 Marya S. Sabir, Mark R. Haussler, Sanchita Mallick et al., "Optimal vitamin D spurs serotonin: 1,25-dihydroxyvitamin D represses serotonin reuptake transport (*SERT*) and degradation (*MAO-A*) gene expression in cultured rat serotonergic neuronal cell lines," *Genes & Nutrition* 13 (2018): 19, doi:10.1186/s12263-018-0605-7.

147 Suvarna Satish Khadilkar, "The Emerging Role of Vitamin D_3 in Women's Health," *Journal of Obstetrics & Gynecology of India* 63, no. 3 (2013): 147–50, doi:10.1007/s13224-013-0420-4.

148 T. L. Clemens, J. S. Adams, S. L. Henderson et al., "Increased skin pigment reduces the capacity of skin to synthesise vitamin D_3," *Lancet* 1 (1982): 74–76, doi:10.1016/s0140-6736(82)90214-8.

149 A. Catharine Ross, Christine L. Taylor, Ann L. Yaktine, and Heather B. Del Valle, eds. *Dietary Reference Intakes for Calcium and Vitamin D* (Washington, D.C.: National Academies Press, 2011).

150 Behzad Heidari and Maryam Beygom Haji Mirghassemi, "Seasonal variations in serum vitamin D according to age and sex," *Capitan Journal of Internal Medicine* 3, no. 4 (2012): 535–40, https://www.ncbi.nlm.nih.gov/pmc/articles/PMC3755860/.

151 Christian Cajochen, Songül Altanay-Ekici, Mirjam Münch et al., "Evidence that the lunar cycle influences human sleep," *Current Biology* 23, no. 15 (2013): 1485–8, doi:10.1016/j.cub.2013.06.029.

152 Justyna M. Wierzbicka, Michal A. Zmijewski, Anna Piotrowska et al., "Bioactive forms of vitamin D selectively stimulate the skin analog of the hypothalamus-pituitary-adrenal axis in human epidermal keratinocytes," *Molecular and Cellular Endocrinology* 437 (2016): 312–22, doi:10.1016/j.mce.2016.08.006.

153 Yoshihiro J. Ono, Akiko Tanabe, Yoko Nakamura et al., "A Low-Testosterone State Associated with Endometrioma Leads to the Apoptosis of Granulosa Cells," *PLoS One* 9, no. 12 (2014), doi:10.1371/journal.pone.0115618.

154 H. A. Bischoff-Ferrari, E. J. Orav, and B. Dawson-Hughes, "Additive benefit of higher testosterone levels and vitamin D plus calcium supplementation in regard to fall risk reduction among older men and women," *Osteoporosis International* 19, no. 9 (2008): 1307–14, doi:10.1007/s00198-008-0573-7.

155 Fabiene Bernardes Castro Vale, Junia Duelli Boroni, Guilherme Geber et al., "Effect of Tribulus Terrestris in the Treatment of Female Sexual Dysfunction and Clitoral Vascularization. Results of a Randomized Study Comparing Two Different Dosage Regimes," *Journal of Sex & Marital Therapy* 47, no. 7 (2021): 696–706, doi:10.1080/0092623X.2021.1938764.

156 Leila Mazaheri Nia, Mina Iravani, Parvin Abedi et al., "Effect of Zinc on Testosterone Levels and Sexual Function of Postmenopausal Women: A Randomized Controlled Trial," *Journal of Sex & Marital Therapy* 47, no. 8 (2021): 804–813, doi:10.1080/0092623X.2021.1957732.

157 Sina Mojaverrostami, Narjes Asghari, Mahsa Khamisabadi et al., "The role of melatonin in polycystic ovary syndrome: A review," *International Journal of Reproductive BioMedicine* 17, no, 12 (2019): 865–82, doi:10.18502/ijrm.v17i12.5789.

158 Sina Mojaverrostami, Narjes Asghari, Mahsa Khamisabadi et al., "The role of melatonin in polycystic ovary syndrome: A review," *International Journal of Reproductive BioMedicine* 17, no, 12 (2019): 865–82, doi:10.18502/ijrm.v17i12.5789.

159 Wen-Huey Wu, Yu-Ping Kang, Nai-Hung Wang et al., "Sesame ingestion affects sex hormones, antioxidant status, and blood lipids in postmenopausal women," *Journal of Nutrition* 136, no. 5 (2006): 1270–5, doi:10.1093/jn/136.5.1270.

160 James R. Roney and Zachary L. Simmons, "Elevated Psychological Stress Predicts Reduced Estradiol Concentrations in Young Women," *Adaptive Human Behavior and Physiology* 1 (2015): 30–40, doi:10.1007/s40750-014-0004-2.

161 Alexandra Acevedo-Rodriguez, Shaila K. Mani, and Robert J. Handa, "Oxytocin and Estrogen Receptor ⬚ in the Brain: A̲ ̲ ̲ ̲ ̲ ̲tiers in Endocrinology* 6 (2015): 160, ̲ ̲ ̲.2015.00160.

1̲ ̲ ̲a̲r̲ ̲ ̲ ̲an Anders, Lori Brotto, Janine Farrell et al., "Associations among physiological and subjective sexual response, sexual desire, and salivary steroid hormones in healthy premenopausal women," *Journal of Sexual Medicine* 6, no. 3 (2009): 739–51, doi:10.1111/j.1743-6109.2008.01123.x.

163 Mohamad Irani and Zaher Merhi, "Role of vitamin D in ovarian physiology and its implication in reproduction: A systematic review," *Fertility and Sterility* 102 (2014), doi:10.1016/j.fertnstert.2014.04.046.

164 Anoma Chandrasekara and Thamilini Josheph Kumar, "Roots and Tuber Crops as Functional Foods: A Review on Phytochemical Constituents and Their Potential Health Benefits," *International Journal of Food Science* (2016), doi:10.1155/2016/3631647.

165 Ewa Walecka-Kapica, Jan Chojnacki, Agnieszka Stepien et al., "Melatonin and Female Hormone Secretion in Postmenopausal Overweight Women," *International Journal of Molecular Sciences* 16, no. 1 (2015): 1030–42, doi:10.3390/ijms16011030.

166 Khatereh Ataei-Almanghadim, Azizeh Farshbaf-Khalili, Ali Reza Ostadrahimi et al., "The effect of oral capsule of curcumin and vitamin E on the hot flashes and anxiety in postmenopausal women: A triple blind randomised controlled trial," *Complementary Therapies in Medicine* 48 (2020), doi:10.1016/j.ctim.2019.102267.

167 B. Raccah-Tebeka, G. Boutet, and G. Plu-Bureau, "Non-hormonal alternatives for the management of menopausal hot flushes. Postmenopausal women management: CNGOF and GEMVi practice guidelines," *Gynécologie Obstétrique Fertilité & Sénologie* 49, no. 5 (2021): 373–93, doi:10.1016/j.gofs.2021.03.020.

168 Mary Lee Barron, "Light Exposure, Melatonin Secretion, and Menstrual Cycle Parameters: An Integrative Review," *Biological Research for Nursing* 9, no. 1 (2007): 49–69, doi:10.1177/1099800407303337.

169 Shilpi Rajoria, Robert Suriano, Perminder Singh Parmar et al., "3,3'-Diindolylmethane Modulates Estrogen Metabolism in Patients with Thyroid Proliferative Disease: A Pilot Study," *Thyroid* 21, no. 3 (2011): 299–304, doi:10.1089/they.2010.0245.

170 Susan J. Jewlings and Douglas S. Kalman, "Curcumin: A Review of Its Effects on Human Health," *Foods* 6, no. 10 (2017): 92, doi:10.3390/foods6100092.

171 Ying Zhang, Hong Cao, Zheng Yu et al., "Curcumin inhibits endometriosis endometrial cells by reducing estradiol production," *Iranian Journal of Reproductive Medicine* 11, no. 5 (2013): 415–22, https://www.ncbi.nlm.nih.gov/pmc/articles/PMC3941414/.

172 Leila Amini, Razieh Chekini, Mohammad Reza Nateghi et al., "The Effect of Combined Vitamin C and Vitamin E

Supplementation on Oxidative Stress Markers in Women with Endometriosis: A Randomized, Triple-Blind Placebo-Controlled Clinical Trial," *Pain Research and Management* (2021), doi:10.1155/2021/5529741.

173 Sina Mojaverrostami, Narjes Asghari, Mahsa Khamisabadi et al., "The role of melatonin in polycystic ovary syndrome: A review," *International Journal of Reproductive BioMedicine* 17, no, 12 (2019): 865–82, doi:10.18502/ijrm.v17i12.5789.

174 Mohaddese Mahboubi, "Evening Primrose (*Oenothera biennis*) Oil in Management of Female Ailments," *Journal of Menopausal Medicine* 25, no. 2 (2019): 74–82, doi:10.6118/jmm.18190.

175 Hirofumi Henmi, Toshiaki Endo, Yoshimitsu Kitajima et al., "Effects of Ascorbic acid supplementation on serum progesterone levels in patients with a luteal phase defect," *Fertility and Sterility* 80, no. 2 (2003): 459–61, doi:10.1015/S0015-0282(03)00567-5.

176 Vincenzo Triggiani, Emilio Tafaro, Vito Angelo Giagulli et al., "Role of iodine, selenium and other micronutrients in thyroid function and disorders," *Endocrine, Metabolic & Immune Disorders–Drug Targets* 9, no. 3 (2009): 277–94, doi:10.2174/187153009789044392.

177 A. Dunaif, "Insulin resistance and the polycystic ovary syndrome: mechanism and implications for pathogenesis," *Endocrine Reviews* 18, no. 6 (1997): 774–800, doi:10.1210/edrv.18.6.0318.

178 "Why Eat Seasonally?" Season Food Guide, https://www.seasonalfoodguide.org/why-eat-seasonally.

179 "Local Food Directories: National Farmers Market Directory," USDA Agricultural Marketing Service, https://www.ams.usda.gov/local-food-directories/farmersmarkets.

180 "Local Food Directories: Community Supported Agriculture (CSA) Directory," USDA Agricultural Marketing Service, https://www.ams.usda.gov/local-food-directories/csas.

181 "Mercury in Fish: A Guide to Protecting Your Family's Health," Natural Resources Defense Council, https://www.nrdc.org/sites/default/files/walletcard.pdf.

182 "Dirty Dozen: EWG's 2021 Shopper's Guide to Pesticides in Produce," Environmental Working Group, https://www.ewg.org/foodnews/dirty-dozen.php.

183 "EWG's Skin Deep®," Environmental Working Group, https://www.ewg.org/skindeep/.

184 "Find an ND," The American Association of Naturopathic Physicians, https://naturopathic.org/search/custom.asp?id=5613.

185 "Find Your ND," Institute for Natural Medicine, https://naturemed.org/find-an-nd/.

186 "Find a Practitioner," The Institute for Functional Medicine, https://www.ifm.org/find-a-practitioner/.

INDEX

A

adrenal glands, 13, 146–147
aging, 29–30
  adjusting eating with, 42
  change in hormones with, 9,
    11, 12
  from chronic stress, 29–30
  and hormone balance/
    imbalance, 13
  and oxidative damage, 43–44
  and skin changes, 138
  and skin microbiome, 23
  and skin pH, 22
  and sun exposure, 137
alcohol, 27, 32–33, 42, 137
Almond Crust, Pumpkin Pie with,
  170
androgens, 12, 141, 142
antioxidants, 77, 137
Apple(s)
  Baked, 190
  Salad, Roasted Brussels
    Sprouts and, 164
Artichoke Soup, Creamy, 203
artificial light, 33
Arugula and Sprouts Bowl,
  Poached Eggs over, 192
Asparagus and Fava Bean Salad,
  198

B

bacteria, 24. see also
  microbiomes
Baked Apples, 190
Baked Quail with Roasted
  Parsnips, 178
balance, 1–3
  of hormones, 6, 7, 9–18, 57,
    134 (see also hormones)
  in meals, for blood sugar
    control, 148
  in microbiomes, 19–24
Barley Porridge with Pears,
  172

Barley Salad with Roasted
  Winter Squash, 177
Bath Salts, Body, 94
Beau Pa's Cookies, 167
beauty, 1–3
  and aging, 138
  defined, 2–3
  natural, 3, 5
  as our natural state, 11
  root causes of, 6–7
  as state of mind, 56–57 (see
    also mindset)
bedtime rituals, 94, 111
Bee Pollen, Kiwi Mint Smoothie
  with, 191
Beet Ginger Smoothie Juice, 174
Berry
  Bliss Smoothie Bowl, 210
  Crisp, Summer, 223
bike riding, 70, 88, 109
bioidentical hormones, 18, 141,
  143, 145–146
birth control
  and gut microbiome, 20,
    140–141
  and hormones, 10, 11, 17, 144
  prescribed for other issues, 7
  and vaginal microbiome, 24
Bison Meatloaf with Garlic
  Broccoli, 181
Black Bean
  Dip, Nut Crackers with, 188
  Soup, Swiss Chard and, 182
Black-Eyed Peas, Summer
  Greens Salad with, 214
blood sugar, 14, 15
body. see also health
  choices affecting, 6
  innate wisdom of, 2
  toxins in, 43
body awareness, 32, 87, 128–129
Body Bath Salts, 94
body fat, 13. see also weight
Body Oil, Cleansing, 228

Body Scrub, Winter, 228
bones, 10–12, 138, 141–142
bowel movements, 140, 147
BPA, 46–47
brain, 26–29
brain fog, 12
Braised Turnips and Greens
  Bowl, 201
breathing, 31–35, 57, 74, 91, 129
Broccoli
  Garlic, Bison Meatloaf with,
    181
  Soup, Creamy, 161
Brussels Sprouts, Roasted, and
  Apple Salad, 164
buddy workouts, 71

C

Cabbage Salmon Salad, 186
caffeine, 32, 33, 137
candle-lighting ritual, 110
cardiovascular system, 10, 13, 14
Carrot Salad, 190
chemical sensitivity/reactivity,
  141
Cherry Chocolate Mousse, 207
Chia
  Face Wash, Honey, Green
    Tea, and, 226
  Ginger Pudding, with
    Pomegranate Seeds, 152
  Oats, Overnight, 152
Chicken
  Free-Range Spring Apricot,
    with Leeks, 202
  with Watercress Wraps, 202
childbirth, 16
Chili, Black Bean Turkey, 162
Chips, Kale, 171
Chive Soup, Spring, 196
Chocolate Mousse Parfait,
  Creamy, 222
Chocolate Truffles, 169
Cinnamon
  Granola, 173

Oat Bites, 168
circadian rhythms, 15, 32–35
Cleanser(s), 77, 95
    Chia, Honey, and Green Tea
        Face Wash, 226
    Cleansing Body Oil, 228
    Jojoba Oil and Yogurt, 232
cleansing oil, 94–95
Coconut
    Ice Cream, 221
    Sauce, Melon with, 224
    Smoothie, Peach Mint, 209
collagen
    aiding production of, 97, 98,
        113
    damage to, 44, 138
    nutrients to boost, 53
    for skin, 14
    slowing loss of, 58
    and stress, 32
Collard Greens
    Pan Seared Scallops over, 194
    White Bean Soup with, 157
community projects, 130
conception, 38, 117
confidence, 135
connection, 16, 17, 30, 70, 92,
    126–127
Cookies, Beau Pa's, 167
cortisol, 13–14, 16–18
    levels of, 135, 141, 148
    and sleep, 32
    and stress, 30
    and sunlight, 37
cosmetic lasers, 98
Creamy Artichoke Soup, 203
Creamy Broccoli Soup, 161
Creamy Chocolate Mousse
    Parfait, 222
Creamy Cilantro Green Pea Soup,
    197
creative activities, 75
Crisp
    Strawberry Rhubarb, 206
    Summer Berry, 223
Cucumber
    Face Mist, Mint, 232
    Salad, 217
Custard, Macadamia Nut, 204
cycles and rhythms, 6. see also

seasonal changes
    circadian rhythms, 15, 32–35
    hormonal, 11, 13–15, 25
    menstrual cycles, 7, 12, 16, 61,
        117, 140, 142–144, 147
    of nature, 7

D
dance, 71
Dandelion Strawberry Bowl with
    Macadamia Nuts, 193
decluttering, 109
deep breathing, 34–35
dehydroepiandrosterone
    (DHEA), 13, 141–142
Deodorant, DIY, 132
detoxification, 139–141
diabetes, 14, 15
digestion
    and aging, 42
    and gut microbiome, 21
    and hormone balance/
        imbalance, 10
    personalizing Natural Beauty
        Reset for, 139–141
    in the spring, 99
dihydrotesterone (DHT), 12
Dip
    Black Bean, Nut Crackers
        with, 188
    Egg, with Veggies, 204
DIY Deodorant, 132
dopamine, 26–27, 30, 117
drinks
    daily servings of liquids, 55
    toxins in, 46–47, 49
    water, 124
dry skin brushing, 113

E
Egg(s)
    Dip, with Veggies, 204
    Poached, over Arugula and
        Sprouts Bowl, 192
Eggplant, Roasted, Quinoa
    Lentil Salad with, 158
elastin, 14, 113
Emerson, Ralph Waldo, 116
emotional issues, 7, 139
Endive Lentil Salad with Shallot

Herb Dressing, 187
endocrine-disrupting chemicals
    (EDCs), 10, 45, 58, 147
energy
    and hormone levels, 10, 12–15,
        17–18, 146–148
    and seasonal resets, 135, 139
    in the summer, 116
    and technology use, 136
environment
    and food production/
        transport, 40
    for good sleep, 33–34
    highly sanitized, 19
    and microbiomes, 19, 21–23
    personalizing Natural Beauty
        Reset for, 135–137
    toxins in, 43–49
epinephrine (adrenaline), 28
estrogen, 11, 13, 38, 117, 142–
    145, 148
exercise. see movement
exfoliating, 77, 96–97, 113, 133

F
Face Mask
    Hydrating Watermelon, 233
    Pumpkin, 227
    Strawberry and Apricot, 231
Face Mist, 131
    Cucumber Mint, 232
Face Oil, Spring, 230
Face Refresher, 230
Face Steam(s), 78
    Herbal, 226
    hydrating, 95
Face Wash, Chia, Honey, and
    Green Tea, 226
facials, 78, 97–98
facial sponge, 133
Fall Harvest Salad, 166
Fall Reset, 60–78
    DIY skincare recipes for,
        226–227
    food for, 62–65
    meal ideas for, 66–68
    mindset for, 73–76
    movement for, 69–73
    recipes for, 151–171
    skincare for, 76–78

fast food, 137
Fava Bean Salad, Asparagus and, 198
fertility, 9–13, 38, 47, 58, 99–100, 145
first-aid kit, 132
fitness classes, 70, 90, 109
Fitzgerald, F. Scott, 60
folate, 39, 80
food(s), 5. see also meal ideas; recipes
  adjusting, as we age, 42
  for all seasons, 53–56
  daily servings of, 54–55
  environmental impact of producing, 40
  for Fall Reset, 62–65
  foundational eating, 53–56
  growing practices for, 39–40
  nutritional status of, 38–42
  preservatives in, 40
  and seasonal changes, 38–42
  sensitivity/reactivity to, 141
  for Spring Reset, 100–102
  for Summer Reset, 117–120
  toxins in, 46–47, 49
  whole vs. processed, 40–42
  for Winter Reset, 80–83
forest bathing, 128
fragrance, 45, 46
Free-Range Spring Apricot Chicken with Leeks, 202
fruits
  daily servings of, 54
  in Fall Reset, 63
  in Spring Reset, 101
  in Summer Reset, 118
  in Winter Reset, 81

G

GABA, 27–28
gardening, 53, 62, 109–111, 129, 136
Garlic Broccoli, Bison Meatloaf with, 181
Garlic Kale, Lime Chili Halibut with, 160
Gazpacho, Summer, 217
gender and sexual identity, 4
genetic expression, 25–26

ghrelin, 15–16, 31
Ginger
  Beet Smoothie Juice, 174
  Chia Pudding, with Pomegranate Seeds, 152
Gingerbread Muffins, Gluten-Free, 189
Goat Feta, Watermelon Salad with Mint and, 211
Golden Mango Smoothie, 211
grains
  daily servings of, 55
  in Fall Reset, 63
  in Summer Reset, 118
  in Winter Reset, 81
Granola, Cinnamon, 173
Green Beans, Pesto, Wild Alaskan Salmon with, 212
Green Goddess Smoothie, 211
Green Pea Soup, Creamy Cilantro, 197
Green Smoothie Juice, Ultimate, 153
gut–brain axis, 26
gut microbiome, 19–21
  and food-growing practices, 39–40
  and gut–brain axis, 26
  leaky gut, 21, 141
  repairing, 141
  and skin microbiome, 21–22
gym workouts, 87

H

hair issues, 142, 147
Halibut
  Lime Chili, with Garlic Kale, 160
  Tacos, with Red Cabbage Slaw, 153
health. see also specific topics
  in the fall, 60, 61, 69
  and gut microbiome, 19–20
  and hormones, 9–18
  and neurotransmitters, 28–29
  regular checkups for, 148
  and seasonal resets, 134
  and skincare products, 44–45, 58–59
  skin conditions, 137

and sleep, 31, 57
and sugar consumption, 41, 42, 47
in the summer, 141
and sun exposure, 137
and time spent in nature, 136
and vaginal microbiome, 23–24
and vitamin D levels, 138
heat-trapping ingredients, 132
herbal steams, 78
  Herbal Face Steam, 226
herbs and spices
  daily servings of, 55
  in Fall Reset, 65
  in Spring Reset, 102
  in Summer Reset, 120
  in Winter Reset, 83
high-fructose corn syrup (HFCS), 47, 148
hiking, 70, 107
home, toxins in the, 47–49
home exercise circuits, 71–72
hormone replacement therapy, 143, 145–146
hormones, 9–18. see also individual hormones
  balance/imbalance of, 6, 7, 9–18, 57, 134
  bioidentical, 18, 141, 143, 145–146
  cortisol, 13–14, 18
  dehydroepiandrosterone, 13
  disrupted by skincare products, 45–46, 58, 59
  estrogen, 11
  in the fall, 61–62
  habits that disrupt, 10
  HPA axis and release of, 26
  importance of, 6–7
  insulin, 14–15
  leptin and ghrelin, 15–16
  melatonin, 15
  and memory or mood, 25
  and neurotransmitters, 26–29
  oxytocin, 16–17
  personalizing Natural Beauty Reset for, 141–148
  progesterone, 12, 18

sex, 4, 38
  and sleep, 32–33
  in the spring, 99–100, 106
  and sugar, 41, 42
  in the summer, 116–117
  and sunlight exposure, 37–38,
    61
  testosterone, 12
  that impact health, 10–18
  thyroid hormones, 12–13,
    17–18
  in the winter, 79–80
Hummus, Spring Onion, with
  Nut Crackers, 208
Hydrating Watermelon Face
  Mask, 233
hydration, 95–96
hygiene habits, 19, 21, 22
hyperthyroidism, 13, 147
hypothalamic-pituitary-adrenal
  (HPA) axis, 26, 58
hypothyroidism, 13, 147

I
Ice Cream, Coconut, 221
immune system
  in the fall, 60, 62
  and gut microbiome, 20
  hormones' effect on, 13
  and seasonal changes, 41
  and skin microbiome,
    21, 23
  and thyroid function, 147
  in the winter, 79
infertility, 142, 147
innate wisdom, 2, 6, 7
insecurity, 1–2
insomnia
  amber-lensed glasses for, 33
  and hormones, 11, 14, 17–18,
    142, 144, 146
  and neurotransmitters, 28
insulin, 14–15
insulin resistance, 147–148
intense workouts, 108

J
Jojoba Oil and Yogurt Cleanser,
  232
journaling, 73–74

K
Kale
  Chips, 171
  Garlic, Lime Chili Halibut
    with, 160
Kiwi Mint Smoothie with Bee
  Pollen, 191

L
Lamb Chops with Mint
  Chutney, 215
laughter, 93–94
lead, 46
leaky gut, 21, 141
leaky skin, 21
Leek(s)
  Free-Range Spring Apricot
    Chicken with, 202
  Pork Chops with Mashed
    Yams and, 179
  Potato Soup, 185
legumes
  in Fall Reset, 64
  in Spring Reset, 101
  in Summer Reset, 119
  in Winter Reset, 82
Lentil
  Endive Salad, with Shallot
    Herb Dressing, 187
  Quinoa Salad, with Roasted
    Eggplant, 158
  Red, Soup, 163
leptin, 15–16, 31, 37, 80
lifestyle, 40
  for good sleep, 32–33
  and neurotransmitters, 26–29
  for optimum hormone levels,
    142, 143, 145, 146
  personalizing Natural Beauty
    Reset for, 135–137
  and signs of aging, 138
  for supporting microbiomes,
    24
light. see also sunlight exposure
  artificial, 33
  in the fall, 75
  from technology screens, 76
  window bathing, 91–92
Lime Chili Halibut with Garlic
  Kale, 160

Lip Balm, Soothing, 229
lip moisturizers, 95
liquids, daily servings of, 55. see
  also drinks

M
Macadamia Nut(s)
  -Crusted Trout with Pineapple
    Chutney, 216
  Custard, 202
  Dandelion Strawberry Bowl
    with, 194
makeup, 115
Mango, Golden, Smoothie, 211
mantra meditation, 74–75
masks, 95
meal ideas. see also recipes
  for Fall Reset, 66–68
  for Spring Reset, 103–105
  for Summer Reset, 121–123
  for Winter Reset, 48–86
meditation, 74–75, 110, 128
melatonin, 15, 17–18, 142–145
  protective role of, 137
  seasonal changes in, 37–38, 80
  and skin, 57
  and sleep, 32, 36, 62
Melon with Coconut Sauce, 222
memory, 13, 25–29
menopause, 11–13, 15, 117,
    141–146
menstrual cycles
  birth control pills to regulate,
    7, 140
  and hormones, 12, 13, 142–
    144, 147
  and seasonal changes, 61, 117
mercury, 46
metabolism
  and hormones, 10, 13, 14, 147
  and seasonal resets, 134
  in the winter, 79, 80
microbiomes, 19–24. see also
    individual microbiomes
  gut, 19–21
  skin, 21–23
  and soil, 39–40, 106
  vaginal, 23–24
microneedling, 97
mindfulness, 57, 128, 143

mindset, 3, 5, 141
  and adrenal function, 146
  for all seasons, 56–57
  for Fall Reset, 73–76
  healthy, 6
  for Spring Reset, 109–111
  for stress reduction, 139
  for Summer Reset, 128–130
  and thyroid function, 147
  for Winter Reset, 90–94
  with yoga, 45
Mint
  Chutney, Lamb Chops with, 215
  Face Mist, Cucumber, 232
  Smoothie, Kiwi with Bee Pollen, 191
  Smoothie, Peach Coconut, 209
  Watermelon Salad, with Goat Feta and, 213
moisturizers, 76, 95, 113–114, 133
mold, 48
mood, 25–30. see also mindset
  and androgen levels, 142
  and artificial light, 33
  and chronic stress, 30
  in the fall, 60, 61, 73
  and hormones, 9–13, 15–18, 146–148
  and movement, 69
  and seasonal resets, 134–135, 139
  in the summer, 116–117
  in the winter, 79
morning workouts, 88–89, 107–108
motivation, 134, 141–142
Mousse, Cherry Chocolate, 207
movement, 5
  for all seasons, 56
  for Fall Reset, 69–73
  and sleep quality, 35
  for Spring Reset, 106–109
  for Summer Reset, 124–128
  for Winter Reset, 86–90
Muffins, Gluten-Free Gingerbread, 187
muscle issues, 12, 141–142, 146

N
natural beauty, 3, 5
Natural Beauty Reset, 3, 17. see also 7-Day Natural Beauty Reset
natural rhythms, 6, 7
nature
  exploring, 130
  health benefits of being in, 106
  reattuning to, 40
  spending time in, 30, 124, 136
neurotransmitters, 26–29. see also specific neurotransmitters
new activities, trying, 111
norepinephrine (noradrenaline), 28
northern hemisphere, 135
Nut(s)
  Crackers, with Black Bean Dip, 188
  daily servings of, 54
  in Fall Reset, 64
  in Spring Reset, 102
  in Summer Reset, 119
  in Winter Reset, 82
nutritional status
  in the fall, 61, 62
  of foods, 38–42, 62
  in the summer, 117
  for vegetarians, 135–136
  and vitamin D deficiency, 138–139
  in the winter, 79–80

O
Oat(s)
  Bites, Cinnamon, 168
  Overnight Chia, 152
oils
  daily servings of, 55
  Face Oil, Spring, 230
  oxidized, 47
  for skin, 113–114
online workouts, 87–88
outdoor bootcamps, 124, 126
Overnight Chia Oats, 152
ovulation, 99, 142
oxidative damage, 43–44, 137

oxybenzone (benzophenone), 45–46, 59
oxytocin, 16–17, 93

P
Pacific Sardines Salad, 196
Pan Seared Scallops over Collard Greens, 194
parabens, 45
Parfait, Creamy Chocolate Mousse, 222
park workouts, 126
Parsley Pesto, Turkey Meatballs with Zucchini Pasta and, 155
Parsnips, Roasted, Baked Quail with, 178
Pasta, Zucchini, Turkey Meatballs with Parsley Pesto and, 155
Peach
  Smoothie, Coconut Mint, 209
  Summer Salad, Tomato and, 18
Pears, Barley Porridge with, 172
perimenopause, 13, 23, 25, 118, 143–146
Persimmon Smoothie Bowl, 173
personalizing the 7-Day Natural Beauty Reset, 134–148
  for digestion and detoxification, 139–141
  for hormone balance, 141–148
  for sleep and stress, 139
  for your lifestyle and environment, 135–137
  for your skin, 137–139
pesticides, 46
Pesto
  Green Beans, Wild Alaskan Salmon with, 212
  Parsley, Turkey Meatballs with Zucchini Pasta and, 155
phytoestrogens, 142–143
Pie, Pumpkin, with Almond Crust, 170
Pineapple Chutney, Macadamia-Crusted Trout with, 216
platelet-rich plasma (PRP) facials, 97–98

Poached Eggs over Arugula and Sprouts Bowl, 192
polychlorinated biphenyls (PCBs), 46
polycyclic aromatic hydrocarbons (PAHs), 47
polycystic ovary syndrome (PCOS), 12, 142, 147–148
Pomegranate Seeds, Ginger Chia Pudding with, 152
Pork Chops with Leeks and Mashed Yams, 179
Porridge, Barley, with Pears, 172
Potato Leek Soup, 185
prayer, 74–75
pregnancy, 11, 25, 47, 117, 138. see also reproduction
preservatives, 40, 45, 46
progesterone, 12, 18, 143–145, 148
progestin, 145
protein
  daily servings of, 54–55
  in Fall Reset, 65
  sources of, 135–136
  in Spring Reset, 102
  in Summer Reset, 120
  in Winter Reset, 83
Pudding, Ginger Chia, with Pomegranate Seeds, 152
Pumpkin
  Face Mask, 227
  Pie, with Almond Crust, 170
  Spice Smoothie, 151

Q
qigong, 71
Quail, Baked, with Roasted Parsnips, 178
Quinoa Lentil Salad with Roasted Eggplant, 158

R
Ratatouille, 218
recipes. see also meal ideas
  for Fall Reset, 151–171
  for skincare, 225–233
  for Spring Reset, 191–208
  for Summer Reset, 209–224
  for Winter Reset, 172–190

recreational drugs, 137
Red Cabbage Slaw, Halibut Tacos with, 153
Red Lentil Soup, 163
reproduction, 99
  birth control, 7, 10, 11, 17, 20, 24, 140–141, 144
  childbirth, 16
  fertility, 9–13, 38, 47, 58, 99–100, 145
  infertility, 142, 147
  ovulation, 99, 142
  pregnancy, 11, 25, 47, 117, 138
Rhubarb Strawberry Crisp, 206
Rumi, 1
running, 88, 107

S
Salad
  Asparagus and Fava Bean, 198
  Barley, with Roasted Winter Squash, 177
  Carrot, 190
  Cucumber, 215
  Endive Lentil, with Shallot Herb Dressing, 187
  Fall Harvest, 166
  Pacific Sardines, 196
  Quinoa Lentil, with Roasted Eggplant, 158
  Roasted Brussels Sprouts and Apple, 164
  Salmon Cabbage, 186
  Spring Greens and Strawberry, 199
  Summer Greens, with Black-Eyed Peas, 214
  Tomato and Peach, 218
  Watermelon, with Mint and Goat Feta, 213
Salmon
  Cabbage Salad, 186
  Wild Alaskan, with Pesto Green Beans, 212
Salsa, Roasted Tomatillo, 224
Sardines, Pacific, Salad, 196
Scallops, Pan Seared, over Collard Greens, 194
seasonal changes, 5, 6, 37–42
  areas without, 135

and hormones, 13–16, 37–38
and natural beauty, 51 (see also 7-Day Natural Beauty Reset)
and sleep, 32
seeds
  daily servings of, 54
  in Fall Reset, 64
  in Spring Reset, 102
  in Summer Reset, 119
  in Winter Reset, 82
self-doubt, 2
serotonin, 28–30, 39, 61, 62, 80, 117
7-Day Natural Beauty Reset, 5, 51
  Fall Reset, 60–78 (see also Fall Reset)
  foods for all seasons, 53–56
  mindset for all seasons, 56–57
  movement for all seasons, 56
  personalizing (see personalizing the 7-Day Natural Beauty Reset)
  resources for, 234
  results of, 134
  skincare for all seasons, 57–59
  Spring Reset, 99–115 (see also Spring Reset)
  Summer Reset, 116–133 (see also Summer Reset)
  Winter Reset, 79–98 (see also Winter Reset)
sex drive, 10, 12, 13, 17, 141–142
sex hormones, 4, 38
Shallot Herb Dressing, Endive Lentil Salad with, 187
simplifying, 110–111
skin, 57–58
  and hormones, 9–14, 17–18, 59, 146–147
  issues with, 7, 21, 137, 138, 141–142
  oxidative damage to, 44 (see also sunlight exposure)
  personalizing Natural Beauty Reset for, 137–139
  pH level of, 22–23, 58
  and seasonal resets, 134–135
  and sleep deprivation, 31–32

and stress management,
29–30, 58
skincare, 5
for all seasons, 57–59
for Fall Reset, 76–78
natural actives in, 23
recipes for, 225–233
sensitivity/reactivity to
products, 141
and skin pH, 22–23
for Spring Reset, 111–115
for Summer Reset, 130–133
toxins in, 44–46, 48–49, 58
for Winter Reset, 94–98
skin microbiome, 21–23
Slaw, Red Cabbage, Halibut
Tacos with, 153
sleep, 31–36, 141
and circadian rhythms, 32–35
and hormone balance/
imbalance, 10–15, 17–18,
146–147
melatonin release during, 15
and mindset, 57
personalizing Natural Beauty
Reset for, 139
and seasonal resets, 135
tips for improving, 35–36
in the winter, 90–91
Smoothie
Golden Mango, 211
Green Goddess, 211
Kiwi Mint, with Bee Pollen,
191
Peach Coconut Mint, 209
Pumpkin Spice, 151
Spring Greens, 191
Smoothie Bowl
Berry Bliss, 210
Persimmon, 173
Smoothie Juice
Beet Ginger, 174
Ultimate Green, 153
social fitness hour, 126–127
Soothing Lip Balm, 229
Soup
Black Bean and Swiss Chard,
182
Creamy Artichoke, 203
Creamy Broccoli, 161

Creamy Cilantro Green Pea,
197
Potato Leek, 185
Red Lentil, 163
Spring Chive, 196
Summer Gazpacho, 217
White Bean, with Collard
Greens, 157
Winter Squash, 184
southern hemisphere, 135
The Spa Dr. skincare, 22, 23, 48,
59, 138
sports, 70, 71, 90, 126
Spring Chive Soup, 196
spring-cleaning, 109, 112–113
Spring Face Oil, 230
Spring Greens
Smoothie, 191
and Strawberry Salad, 199
Spring Onion Hummus with
Nut Crackers, 208
Spring Reset, 99–115
DIY skincare recipes for,
230–231
food for, 100–102
meal ideas for, 103–105
mindset for, 109–111
movement for, 106–109
recipes for, 191–208
skincare for, 111–115
Sprouts and Arugula Bowl,
Poached Eggs over, 192
Steinbeck, John, 79
Stew, Warming Venison, 175
Strawberry
Dandelion Bowl, with
Macadamia Nuts, 194
Face Mask, Apricot and, 231
Rhubarb Crisp, 206
Salad, Spring Greens and,
199
stress, 141
adrenal, 13
aging from, 29–30
and hormone balance/
imbalance, 13, 14, 16
managing, 57
and mood, 30
and neurochemical imbalance,
26

personalizing Natural Beauty
Reset for, 139
and the skin, 29–30, 58
in the winter, 80
stretching, 108, 127–128
sugar, 41–42, 47, 137, 148
Summer Berry Crisp, 223
Summer Gazpacho, 217
Summer Greens Salad with
Black-Eyed Peas, 214
Summer Reset, 116–133
DIY skincare recipes for,
231–233
food for, 117–120
meal ideas for, 121–123
mindset for, 128–130
movement for, 124–128
recipes for, 209–224
skincare for, 130–133
Summer Squash Tacos, 219
sunlight exposure
damage from, 44, 137
and hormones, 36–38, 61
and seasonal eating, 38–39
in the summer, 117, 124, 130,
131
for vitamin D production,
138
in the winter, 91–92
sunscreens, 45–46, 58–59, 77,
114, 124, 131
sweeteners, 55, 148. see also
sugar
sweets
in Fall Reset, 65
in Spring Reset, 102
in Summer Reset, 120
in Winter Reset, 83
swimming, 109, 127
Swiss Chard, Soup, Black Bean
and, 182

T
Tacos
Halibut, with Red Cabbage
Slaw, 153
Summer Squash, 219
tai chi, 71
technology, 6, 33, 136
telomeres, 29, 44

testosterone, 12, 13, 61–62, 69, 141, 142
thyroid hormones, 12–13, 17–18, 38, 61, 80, 147
thyroxine (T4), 12–13, 61, 147
tobacco use, 137
Tomatillo, Roasted, Salsa, 224
Tomato and Peach Summer Salad, 218
touch, 16, 93
toxins, 43–49
    in food and drinks, 46–47, 49
    in the home and workplace, 47–49
    perspiring to eliminate, 45
    reducing exposure to, 48–49
    in skincare, 44–46, 48–49, 58
trauma, 139
triiodothyronine (T3), 12–13, 61, 80, 147
Trout, Macadamia-Crusted, with Pineapple Chutney, 216
Truffles, Chocolate, 169
Turkey
    Chili, Black Bean, 162
    Meatballs, with Parsley Pesto and Zucchini Pasta, 155
Turnips, Braised, and Greens Bowl, 201

U
Ultimate Green Smoothie Juice, 153
urban environments, 136

V
vaginal dryness, 142
vaginal microbiome, 17, 23–24

vegans, 135–136
vegetables
    daily servings of, 54
    in Fall Reset, 64
    in Spring Reset, 101
    in Summer Reset, 119
    in Winter Reset, 82
vegetarians, 135–136
Veggies, Egg Dip with, 204
Venison Stew, Warming, 175
vitamin D, 138–139
    for estrogen production, 143
    in the fall, 61
    seasonal changes in, 38
    from sun exposure, 117, 136–138
    testing for, 139
    in the winter, 79, 91–92

W
walking, 72, 73, 88, 107
walking meditation, 110
Warming Venison Stew, 175
water activities, 127
Watercress Wraps, Chicken with, 202
Watermelon
    Hydrating Face Mask, 233
    Salad, with Mint and Goat Feta, 213
weight, 2
    and artificial light, 33
    and hormone levels, 10, 13–18, 146, 147
    and sleep deprivation, 31
White Bean Soup with Collard Greens, 157
Wild Alaskan Salmon with Pesto Green Beans, 212

Williams, Robin, 99
window bathing, 91–92
Winter Body Scrub, 228
Winter Reset, 79–98
    DIY skincare recipes for, 228–229
    food for, 80–83
    meal ideas for, 48–86
    mindset for, 90–94
    movement for, 86–90
    recipes for, 172–188
    skincare for, 94–98
Winter Squash
    Roasted, Barley Salad with, 177
    Soup, 184
workplace, toxins in the, 47–49

Y
Yams
    Mashed, Pork Chops with Leeks and, 179
    wild, 143
yard work, 72
yoga, 56, 72, 74–75, 89–91, 107, 124

Z
Zucchini Pasta, Turkey Meatballs with Parsley Pesto and, 155

ABOUT
THE AUTHOR

Dr. Trevor Cates is author of the *USA Today* bestselling book *Clean Skin from Within* and founder of The Spa Dr. natural skincare line. She received her medical degree from the National University of Natural Medicine in 2000 and was the first woman licensed as a naturopathic doctor in the state of California. To complement her naturopathic medicine training, she obtained a master's degree in Spiritual Psychology from the University of Santa Monica in 2013.

She was the doctor in several world-renowned spas in Park City, Utah, and continues to help patients from around the world with a focus on women's health, skin, and hormones. She has been featured on various TV shows, including *The Doctors* and *Extra TV*. Dr. Cates is host of the *Hormones, Health, and Harmony* docuseries, *The Woman's Dr.* podcast, and the public television special *Younger Skin from Within*.

Dr. Cates's goal is to inspire and empower women to find the keys to harmonize their hormones and reveal their natural beauty. That beauty has always been there—sometimes we just need a guide to help illuminate the path.